KIDNEY DISEASE DIET COOKBOOK FOR WOMEN

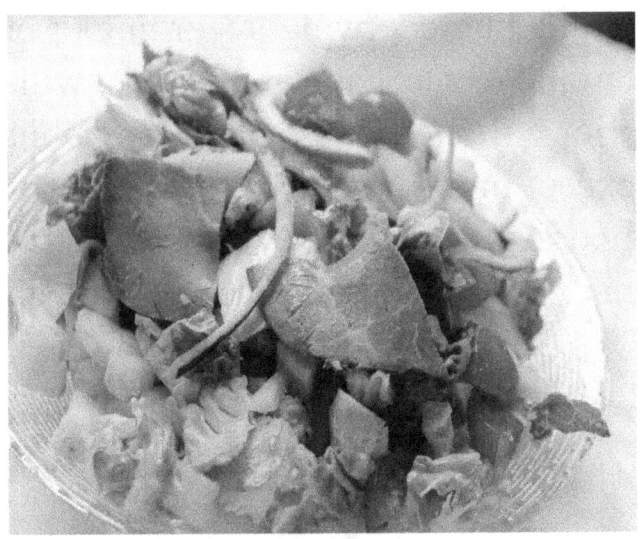

Your Complete Guide to Delicious and Nutritious Recipes to Manage Chronic Kidney Diseases

Tina Feldman

Copyright © Tina Feldman 2024

All rights reserved. No part of this publication may be reproduced, distributed, or transmitted in any form or by any means, including photocopying, recording or other electronic or mechanical methods, without the prior written permission of the publisher, except in the case of brief quotations embodied in critical reviews and certain other non-commercial uses permitted by copyright law.

Table of Contents

INTRODUCTION 9

Part 1: Unveiling Kidney Health for Women 11

    Delving into Kidney Anatomy and Function 11

    Exploring Common Types and Causes of Kidney Disease 13

    Early Symptom Recognition for Women 15

    Unraveling Risk Factors of Kidney Disease 18

    Proactive Prevention Strategies for Women 21

Part 2: Navigating a Kidney-Friendly Diet 25

    Essential Nutritional Requirements for Optimal Kidney Health 25

    Mastering Sodium Intake for Kidney Patients 29

    Achieving Balance in Potassium and Phosphorus Management 32

    Understanding Protein Consumption's Impact on Kidney Functions 35

    Hydration and Fluid Control Essentials 39

    Creating Your Kidney-Friendly Kitchen 44

    Smart Meal Planning Tips 47

Part 3: Staying Active for Healthy Kidney 52

    Harnessing the Benefits of Regular Exercise for Kidney Health 52

Safe and Effective Workouts Tailored for Women with Kidney Diseases 56

Incorporating Movement into Daily Life 62

Exploring the Vital Role of Sleep in Kidney Function 66

PART 4: HEALTHY AND DELICIOUS RECIPES 71

Breakfast Recipes 71

Vegetable Omelette 71

Greek Yogurt Parfait 72

Spinach and Mushroom Frittata 72

Quinoa Breakfast Bowl 73

Avocado Toast with Poached Egg 74

Banana Walnut Smoothie 74

Cottage Cheese and Fruit Bowl 75

Whole Grain Pancakes with Berries 76

Egg and Veggie Breakfast Burrito 77

Mediterranean Breakfast Bowl 78

Blueberry Almond Chia Pudding 78

Turkey and Veggie Breakfast Wrap 79

Sweet Potato and Black Bean Breakfast Hash 80

Apple Cinnamon Overnight Oats 81

Lunch Recipes 82

Grilled Lemon Herb Chicken Salad 82

Quinoa and Black Bean Stuffed Bell Peppers......... 83

Salmon and Asparagus Quiche............................... 84

Vegetarian Lentil Soup 85

Tuna Salad Lettuce Wraps....................................... 86

Mushroom and Spinach Whole Grain Pasta 87

Chickpea and Avocado Salad................................... 88

Turkey and Veggie Wrap 88

Sesame Ginger Tofu Stir-Fry.................................... 89

Caprese Quinoa Salad 90

Vegetable and Bean Chili 91

Eggplant and Tomato Pasta 92

Turkey and Bean Chili... 93

Mediterranean Chickpea Salad 94

Dinner Recipes 95

Baked Lemon Herb Salmon 95

Vegetable Stir-Fry with Tofu 96

Baked Chicken and Vegetable Casserole 97

Turkey and Vegetable Quinoa Bowl....................... 98

Eggplant Parmesan... 99

Vegetarian Lentil Curry 100

Grilled Chicken Caesar Salad................................ 101

Turkey Meatball and Vegetable Skewers 102

Stuffed Bell Peppers with Quinoa and Black Beans 104
Mediterranean Grilled Vegetable Platter 105
Sautéed Shrimp with Garlic and Spinach 106
Teriyaki Tofu Stir-Fry 106
Lemon Garlic Chicken with Roasted Vegetables .. 107
Salmon and Asparagus Foil Packets 108

Dessert Recipes 110

Berry Parfait 110
Frozen Banana Bites 110
Coconut Chia Pudding 111
Baked Apple with Cinnamon 112
Yogurt Bark with Berries 112
Peanut Butter Banana Smoothie 113
Frozen Yogurt Bark with Mango 114
Blueberry Oatmeal Cookies 114
Chocolate Avocado Mousse 115
Cinnamon Baked Apples 116
Peach Sorbet 117
Chia Seed Pudding with Strawberries 118
Watermelon Mint Salad 118
Mixed Berry Smoothie Bowl 119

Pineapple Coconut Ice Pops 120

Snacks Recipes 120

   Cucumber Hummus Bites 120

   Greek Yogurt with Berries and Almonds 121

   Rice Cake with Avocado and Tomato 122

   Edamame Salad 122

   Caprese Skewers 123

   Turkey and Cheese Roll-Ups 124

   Fruit Salad with Mint 124

   Vegetable Crudité with Yogurt Dip 125

   Stuffed Celery Sticks 125

   Tuna Salad Lettuce Wraps 126

   Quinoa and Vegetable Stuffed Bell Peppers 127

   Cottage Cheese with Pineapple 128

   Spinach and Feta Stuffed Mushrooms 128

   Apple Slices with Almond Butter 129

   Oatmeal Raisin Energy Bites 130

Smoothies Recipes 130

   Berry Blast Smoothie 130

   Green Goddess Smoothie 131

   Banana Almond Smoothie 132

   Tropical Paradise Smoothie 132

Berry Spinach Protein Smoothie 133

Peachy Keen Smoothie.. 134

Cherry Vanilla Smoothie....................................... 135

Minty Pineapple Smoothie................................... 135

Carrot Cake Smoothie 136

Citrus Sunshine Smoothie 137

Chocolate Peanut Butter Smoothie 137

Vanilla Berry Smoothie... 138

Mango Coconut Smoothie 139

Pomegranate Blueberry Smoothie...................... 139

Avocado Kale Smoothie 140

BONUS 141

Shopping list 141

CONCLUSION 149

INTRODUCTION

Welcome to the Kidney Disease Diet Cookbook for Women, a comprehensive guide designed to support women in managing their kidney health through delicious and nutritious recipes. This cookbook is tailored specifically for women who are navigating the challenges of kidney disease and seeking ways to optimize their dietary choices to promote overall wellness.

Kidney disease presents unique challenges, impacting not only physical health but also quality of life. For women, managing kidney disease involves not only addressing the physical aspects but also considering the emotional and social implications that come with it. Whether you're newly diagnosed or have been living with kidney disease for some time, this cookbook is here to provide you with practical guidance, flavorful recipes, and essential nutritional information to support your journey towards better kidney health.

Understanding the importance of a kidney-friendly diet is fundamental to managing kidney disease effectively. This cookbook aims to empower women with the knowledge and resources they need to make informed dietary choices that align with their individual health needs. From managing sodium intake to balancing potassium and phosphorus levels, each recipe in this cookbook is carefully crafted to prioritize kidney health without compromising on taste or satisfaction.

In addition to a diverse array of recipes, this cookbook also includes valuable insights into kidney anatomy and function, common types and causes of kidney disease, early symptom recognition, risk factors, and proactive prevention strategies. Furthermore, it offers practical tips on meal planning, navigating the grocery store, and creating a kidney-friendly kitchen environment.

As women, I understand the importance of nurturing our bodies and taking proactive steps towards better health. With this cookbook as your guide, you'll discover a wealth of delicious recipes that nourish the body, tantalize the taste buds, and support your journey towards optimal kidney health. Whether you're cooking for yourself, your family, or loved ones, these recipes are sure to inspire and delight, making every meal a celebration of health and vitality.

Here's to embracing a kidney-friendly lifestyle and savoring the joy of wholesome, flavorful meals that nourish both body and soul. Let's embark on this culinary journey together, one delicious dish at a time.

Part 1: Unveiling Kidney Health for Women

Delving into Kidney Anatomy and Function

Understanding the intricate workings of the kidneys is essential for women seeking to optimize their kidney health. The kidneys, two bean-shaped organs located on either side of the spine, play a pivotal role in filtering waste products and excess fluids from the bloodstream to produce urine. Beyond this vital function, the kidneys also regulate electrolyte levels, blood pressure, and red blood cell production, making them indispensable for overall well-being.

Anatomy of the Kidneys:
The kidneys consist of several distinct structures, each contributing to their efficient function. The renal cortex, renal medulla, and renal pelvis comprise the main regions of the kidney. Within these regions, nephrons, the functional units of the kidney, play a critical role in filtration. Nephrons filter blood, reabsorb essential nutrients and electrolytes, and excrete waste products to maintain fluid and electrolyte balance.

Function of the Kidneys:
Filtration: Blood enters the kidneys through the renal arteries, where it undergoes filtration in the nephrons. Waste products, toxins, and excess fluids are removed from the blood, while essential substances like glucose, amino acids, and electrolytes are retained.

Reabsorption: After filtration, the nephrons reabsorb essential nutrients and electrolytes, such as sodium, potassium, and calcium, back into the bloodstream to maintain proper balance.

Secretion: In addition to filtration and reabsorption, the kidneys also secrete hormones and enzymes that regulate blood pressure, red blood cell production (via erythropoietin), and calcium metabolism (via calcitriol).

Gender-Specific Considerations:
Women may face unique challenges related to kidney health, particularly during pregnancy. Pregnancy increases the workload on the kidneys, as they must filter waste products not only for the mother but also for the developing fetus. Additionally, hormonal changes during pregnancy can affect kidney function and increase the risk of conditions like preeclampsia, a serious complication characterized by high blood pressure and protein in the urine.

Significance for Women's Health:
Understanding kidney anatomy and function is crucial for women to recognize potential signs of kidney disease and take proactive steps to maintain kidney health. Awareness of risk factors such as diabetes, high blood pressure, obesity, and family history can empower women to make informed lifestyle choices and seek timely medical intervention when needed.

Exploring Common Types and Causes of Kidney Disease

Kidney disease encompasses a range of conditions that affect the structure and function of the kidneys, posing significant health challenges for women worldwide. Understanding the common types and underlying causes of kidney disease is essential for early detection, timely intervention, and effective management.

Chronic Kidney Disease (CKD):
1. Definition: CKD is a progressive condition characterized by the gradual loss of kidney function over time. It is a leading cause of kidney failure and can significantly impact overall health and quality of life.
2. Causes: Common causes of CKD include diabetes, high blood pressure (hypertension), glomerulonephritis (inflammation of the kidney's filtering units), and polycystic kidney disease (a genetic disorder characterized by the growth of cysts in the kidneys).
3. Risk Factors: Women with diabetes, hypertension, obesity, a family history of kidney disease, or a history of kidney infections are at increased risk of developing CKD. Age, smoking, and certain medications can also contribute to the risk.

Acute Kidney Injury (AKI):

1. Definition: AKI is a sudden and temporary loss of kidney function, often occurring in response to severe illness, injury, or medical interventions.
2. Causes: AKI can result from conditions such as severe infection (sepsis), dehydration, kidney obstruction, medications (such as certain antibiotics or contrast dyes used in imaging tests), and autoimmune diseases.
3. Risk Factors: Women with pre-existing health conditions, older adults, and those undergoing surgical procedures are at increased risk of developing AKI. Additionally, certain medications and herbal supplements may increase the susceptibility to AKI.

Polycystic Kidney Disease (PKD):
1. Definition: PKD is an inherited disorder characterized by the growth of fluid-filled cysts in the kidneys, leading to kidney enlargement and impaired function over time.
2. Causes: PKD is primarily caused by genetic mutations that disrupt the normal development of kidney tissue. It can be inherited in an autosomal dominant or autosomal recessive pattern.
3. Risk Factors: Women with a family history of PKD are at increased risk of developing the condition. Other risk factors include age, gender (PKD affects women and men equally), and certain genetic factors.

Glomerulonephritis:
1. Definition: Glomerulonephritis refers to inflammation of the glomeruli, the tiny blood

vessels in the kidneys responsible for filtering waste and excess fluids from the blood.
2. Causes: Glomerulonephritis can be caused by infections (such as strep throat or viral infections), autoimmune diseases (such as lupus or IgA nephropathy), and certain medications or toxins.
3. Risk Factors: Women with autoimmune diseases, chronic infections, or a history of certain medications are at increased risk of developing glomerulonephritis.

Early Symptom Recognition for Women

Recognizing the early symptoms of kidney disease is paramount for women's health, as early detection can lead to timely intervention and improved outcomes. Kidney disease often progresses silently, with symptoms becoming apparent only in later stages when significant damage has already occurred. Therefore, understanding the subtle signs of kidney dysfunction is essential for women to take proactive measures to protect their kidney health.

Changes in Urination Patterns:
1. Increased Urination: Women may notice an increase in the frequency of urination, particularly during the night (nocturia). This can occur as the kidneys struggle to filter waste and excess fluid from the bloodstream.
2. Decreased Urination: Conversely, some women may experience a decrease in urine output, known as oliguria. This can indicate reduced kidney function and impaired filtration.

Presence of Blood in Urine (Hematuria):
Women may observe blood in their urine, which can manifest as pink, red, or cola-colored urine. Hematuria can result from various underlying causes, including urinary tract infections, kidney stones, or inflammation of the kidney's filtering units (glomerulonephritis).

Swelling (Edema):
Edema, or swelling, commonly affects the hands, feet, ankles, and face in individuals with kidney disease. This occurs due to the retention of excess fluid and sodium in the body, often resulting from impaired kidney function.

Fatigue and Weakness:
Chronic kidney disease can lead to anemia, a condition characterized by a deficiency of red blood cells or hemoglobin in the blood. Anemia can cause fatigue, weakness, and difficulty concentrating, significantly impacting a woman's quality of life and daily activities.

Persistent Hypertension (High Blood Pressure):
Uncontrolled hypertension is both a cause and a consequence of kidney disease. Women with kidney dysfunction may experience persistent high blood pressure, which can further exacerbate kidney damage and increase the risk of cardiovascular complications.

Unexplained Weight Loss or Poor Appetite:
Individuals with advanced kidney disease may experience unintended weight loss or a decrease in appetite. This can result from metabolic changes, electrolyte imbalances,

and alterations in taste perception associated with kidney dysfunction.

Skin Rash or Itching (Pruritus):
Pruritus, or persistent itching, can occur in women with kidney disease due to the buildup of waste products and toxins in the bloodstream. Itching may be particularly noticeable in the absence of visible skin lesions.

Muscle Cramps and Bone Pain:
Electrolyte imbalances, such as elevated potassium levels (hyperkalemia), can cause muscle cramps and weakness. Additionally, kidney disease can lead to mineral and bone disorders, contributing to bone pain and increased fracture risk.

Nausea and Vomiting:
Women with kidney disease may experience gastrointestinal symptoms such as nausea, vomiting, and loss of appetite. These symptoms can result from the accumulation of uremic toxins in the bloodstream, affecting digestive function.

Changes in Mental Acuity:
Advanced kidney disease can impair cognitive function, leading to confusion, difficulty concentrating, and memory problems. These neurological symptoms, known as uremic encephalopathy, can significantly impact a woman's daily functioning and quality of life.

It is essential for women to pay attention to these early warning signs and consult with a healthcare professional if they experience persistent or concerning symptoms. Early detection and management of kidney disease are key to preserving kidney function, preventing complications, and promoting overall health and well-being

Unraveling Risk Factors of Kidney Disease

Understanding the risk factors associated with kidney disease is crucial for women to identify potential threats to their kidney health and take proactive steps to mitigate them. While some risk factors are modifiable through lifestyle changes and medical intervention, others, such as genetics and age, may be beyond individual control. By unraveling these risk factors, women can empower themselves to make informed decisions and prioritize kidney health in their overall wellness journey.

Diabetes Mellitus:
Diabetes is one of the leading causes of kidney disease, known as diabetic nephropathy. High blood sugar levels over time can damage the small blood vessels in the kidneys, impairing their ability to filter waste and regulate fluid balance. Women with diabetes, particularly type 1 or type 2 diabetes, are at increased risk of developing kidney disease.

Hypertension (High Blood Pressure):

Chronic hypertension is a significant risk factor for kidney disease, as it can cause damage to the blood vessels and structures within the kidneys. Women with uncontrolled high blood pressure are more likely to experience kidney damage and progressive loss of kidney function over time.

Obesity:
Excess body weight, especially visceral fat around the abdomen, is associated with an increased risk of kidney disease. Obesity contributes to metabolic disturbances, insulin resistance, and inflammation, all of which can promote kidney damage and dysfunction in women.

Family History of Kidney Disease:
Genetics plays a significant role in determining an individual's susceptibility to kidney disease. Women with a family history of kidney disease, particularly close relatives such as parents or siblings, may have an elevated risk of developing similar conditions, including polycystic kidney disease, glomerulonephritis, or other inherited disorders.

Age:
Aging is a natural risk factor for kidney disease, as kidney function tends to decline gradually with age. Women over the age of 60 are at increased risk of developing chronic kidney disease (CKD) and other age-related kidney conditions due to physiological changes in kidney structure and function.

Smoking and Tobacco Use:
Smoking is a modifiable risk factor that can accelerate kidney damage and increase the risk of kidney disease in women. Tobacco smoke contains toxins and carcinogens

that can impair blood flow to the kidneys, promote inflammation, and exacerbate existing kidney conditions.

Cardiovascular Disease:
Women with pre-existing cardiovascular conditions, such as coronary artery disease, heart failure, or peripheral vascular disease, are at higher risk of developing kidney disease. Cardiovascular risk factors such as atherosclerosis, dyslipidemia, and inflammation can contribute to kidney damage and compromise renal function over time.

Autoimmune Diseases:
Autoimmune diseases, such as lupus (systemic lupus erythematosus) or vasculitis, can cause inflammation and damage to the kidneys, leading to autoimmune kidney diseases like lupus nephritis. Women with autoimmune conditions are at increased risk of kidney complications and require vigilant monitoring and management.

Urinary Tract Infections (UTIs):
Recurrent urinary tract infections, especially when left untreated or inadequately managed, can lead to kidney damage and scarring. Women are more prone to UTIs due to anatomical factors, making UTIs a potential risk factor for kidney disease in this population.

Medications and Toxins:
Certain medications, such as nonsteroidal anti-inflammatory drugs (NSAIDs), certain antibiotics, and contrast agents used in imaging studies, can cause kidney damage and impair renal function, particularly with

prolonged or excessive use. Women should use medications cautiously and under medical supervision to minimize the risk of kidney-related complications.

Proactive Prevention Strategies for Women

Empowering women with proactive prevention strategies is essential for reducing the incidence and progression of kidney disease. By adopting lifestyle modifications, managing chronic conditions effectively, and prioritizing kidney health, women can take control of their well-being and lower their risk of developing kidney-related complications. Here are key proactive prevention strategies for women:

Maintain a Healthy Lifestyle:
1. Balanced Diet: Embrace a diet rich in fruits, vegetables, whole grains, lean proteins, and healthy fats. Limit processed foods, saturated fats, cholesterol, and refined sugars. Adopting a kidney-friendly diet low in sodium, phosphorus, and potassium can help preserve kidney function.

2. Regular Exercise: Engage in regular physical activity, such as walking, jogging, swimming, or yoga, to promote cardiovascular health and maintain a healthy weight. Aim for at least 150 minutes of moderate-intensity exercise per week, as recommended by health guidelines.
3. Manage Weight: Maintain a healthy weight through a combination of balanced nutrition and regular exercise. Obesity is a significant risk factor for kidney disease, so achieving and maintaining a healthy body weight is crucial for kidney health.
4. Stay Hydrated: Drink an adequate amount of water throughout the day to support kidney function and prevent dehydration. Aim for at least 8-10 cups of fluids daily, adjusting based on individual needs and activity levels.
5. Limit Alcohol and Tobacco: Reduce alcohol consumption and avoid tobacco use, as both can contribute to kidney damage and impair overall health.

Monitor and Manage Chronic Conditions:
1. Control Blood Sugar: If diagnosed with diabetes, manage blood sugar levels through medication, lifestyle modifications, and regular monitoring. Keeping blood glucose levels within target ranges can help prevent diabetic nephropathy and slow the progression of kidney disease.
2. Manage Hypertension: Maintain blood pressure within recommended targets (typically < 130/80 mmHg) through lifestyle changes and medication if necessary. Monitoring blood pressure regularly and adhering to treatment plans can help prevent hypertension-related kidney damage.

3. Manage Lipid Levels: Control cholesterol and triglyceride levels through dietary changes, exercise, and medication if prescribed. Elevated lipid levels can contribute to atherosclerosis and increase the risk of kidney disease and cardiovascular complications.
4. Regular Medical Check-ups: Schedule regular health screenings and check-ups with a healthcare provider to monitor kidney function, blood pressure, blood sugar, and lipid levels. Early detection of abnormalities allows for timely intervention and disease management.

Avoid Nephrotoxic Substances:
1. Use Medications Wisely: Take medications only as prescribed by a healthcare provider and avoid over-the-counter medications, herbal supplements, or alternative therapies that may harm kidney function. Discuss potential nephrotoxic effects of medications with a healthcare provider.
2. Avoid Environmental Toxins: Minimize exposure to environmental toxins, pollutants, and chemicals that may negatively impact kidney health. Use protective gear when handling toxic substances and follow safety guidelines in the workplace and at home.

Promote Overall Wellness:
1. Manage Stress: Practice stress-reduction techniques such as mindfulness, meditation, deep breathing exercises, or yoga to promote mental and emotional well-being. Chronic stress can contribute to hypertension and cardiovascular disease, which are risk factors for kidney disease.

2. Get Adequate Sleep: Prioritize quality sleep by maintaining a consistent sleep schedule, creating a relaxing sleep environment, and practicing good sleep hygiene habits. Aim for 7-8 hours of restorative sleep per night to support overall health and well-being.

Educate and Advocate for Kidney Health:
1. Raise Awareness: Educate yourself and others about the importance of kidney health, risk factors for kidney disease, and proactive prevention strategies. Advocate for policies and initiatives that support kidney health promotion, early detection, and access to care.
2. Support Research: Participate in clinical trials, fundraisers, or advocacy efforts aimed at advancing kidney disease research, treatment options, and patient support services. By actively engaging in the kidney health community, women can contribute to ongoing efforts to improve outcomes and quality of life for individuals affected by kidney disease.

Part 2: Navigating a Kidney-Friendly Diet

Essential Nutritional Requirements for Optimal Kidney Health

Maintaining optimal kidney health requires careful attention to dietary choices, as nutrition plays a critical role in supporting kidney function and preventing complications associated with kidney disease. Navigating a kidney-friendly diet involves understanding the essential nutritional requirements that promote kidney health while minimizing the risk of further damage. Here are key components of a kidney-friendly diet:

Controlled Protein Intake:
1. Protein is essential for overall health, but excessive protein consumption can strain the kidneys, especially in individuals with kidney disease. Aim for moderate protein intake, with a focus on high-quality sources such as lean meats, poultry, fish, eggs, dairy products, and plant-based proteins like beans, lentils, and tofu.
2. Consult with a healthcare provider or registered dietitian to determine the appropriate amount of protein based on individual needs, kidney function, and stage of kidney disease. Protein needs may vary depending on factors such as age, gender, body weight, and level of physical activity.

Sodium Restriction:
1. Limiting sodium (salt) intake is crucial for managing fluid balance and blood pressure, both of which are key factors in preserving kidney

function. Excess sodium can lead to fluid retention and hypertension, placing additional strain on the kidneys.
2. Choose low-sodium or sodium-free alternatives to processed and packaged foods, which are often high in sodium. Use herbs, spices, lemon juice, and other flavorings to enhance the taste of meals without adding extra salt. Aim to consume less than 2,300 milligrams of sodium per day, or even less if advised by a healthcare provider.

Balanced Potassium Levels:
1. Potassium is an electrolyte that plays a vital role in muscle function, nerve transmission, and fluid balance. However, individuals with kidney disease may experience difficulty regulating potassium levels, leading to hyperkalemia (high potassium levels) or hypokalemia (low potassium levels).
2. Choose potassium-rich foods in moderation and monitor potassium intake closely, especially if kidney function is compromised. High-potassium foods include bananas, oranges, potatoes, tomatoes, spinach, and avocados. Cooking methods such as boiling or leaching can help reduce potassium content in certain foods.
3. Work with a healthcare provider or registered dietitian to develop a personalized meal plan that balances potassium intake while meeting nutritional needs.

Phosphorus Management:
1. Phosphorus is a mineral that works in tandem with calcium to maintain bone health and cellular function. However, individuals with kidney

disease often experience elevated phosphorus levels, which can contribute to mineral and bone disorders (renal osteodystrophy) and cardiovascular complications.
2. Limit phosphorus-rich foods such as dairy products, processed meats, nuts, seeds, and certain grains. Choose lower-phosphorus alternatives and consider using phosphate binders as prescribed by a healthcare provider to reduce phosphorus absorption from food.
3. Opt for fresh, unprocessed foods whenever possible, as they tend to have lower phosphorus content compared to processed and convenience foods.

Fluid Control:
1. Proper fluid management is essential for individuals with kidney disease, particularly those experiencing fluid retention (edema) or undergoing dialysis. Monitoring fluid intake helps maintain fluid balance, prevent dehydration, and alleviate strain on the kidneys.
2. Limit fluid intake based on individual fluid restrictions recommended by a healthcare provider or renal dietitian. Adjust fluid intake according to urine output, thirst, and activity level, while avoiding excessive fluid consumption.
3. Choose thirst-quenching beverages such as water, herbal teas, and homemade fruit-infused water over sugary drinks, sodas, and caffeinated beverages, which can contribute to fluid overload and electrolyte imbalances.

Optimal Nutrient Intake:

1. Ensure adequate intake of essential nutrients such as vitamins, minerals, and antioxidants to support overall health and well-being. Incorporate a variety of nutrient-dense foods into your diet, including fruits, vegetables, whole grains, and healthy fats.
2. Consider taking nutritional supplements as recommended by a healthcare provider or registered dietitian to address specific nutrient deficiencies or meet increased nutritional needs associated with kidney disease, such as vitamin D, iron, or B vitamins.

Individualized Meal Planning:
1. Work with a registered dietitian specializing in renal nutrition to develop a personalized meal plan tailored to your specific dietary needs, preferences, and health goals. A renal dietitian can provide guidance on portion control, food choices, cooking methods, and dining out while managing kidney disease.
2. Monitor dietary changes and their impact on kidney function, blood pressure, blood sugar, and other relevant health markers. Adjust your meal plan as needed in collaboration with your healthcare team to optimize kidney health and overall nutritional status.

Mastering Sodium Intake for Kidney Patients

Sodium intake plays a crucial role in managing kidney disease, as excessive sodium consumption can exacerbate fluid retention, elevate blood pressure, and strain the kidneys. Mastering sodium intake is essential for kidney patients to maintain fluid balance, control blood pressure, and slow the progression of kidney damage. Here's a detailed exploration of strategies to effectively manage sodium intake for kidney patients:

Understanding Sodium's Impact on Kidney Health:
1. Sodium, a component of salt, is an electrolyte that regulates fluid balance and helps maintain blood pressure. However, excessive sodium intake can lead to fluid retention and hypertension, both of which are detrimental to kidney function.
2. In individuals with compromised kidney function, the kidneys may struggle to excrete excess sodium, leading to sodium accumulation in the bloodstream. This can contribute to edema (fluid retention), exacerbate hypertension, and further impair kidney function.

Recommended Sodium Intake:
1. The recommended daily sodium intake for individuals with kidney disease varies depending on factors such as stage of kidney disease, blood pressure control, and presence of other comorbidities. However, in general, most kidney patients are advised to limit their sodium intake to less than 2,300 milligrams per day, with further restriction to 1,500 milligrams or less for those with hypertension or advanced kidney disease.

2. Working with a healthcare provider or registered dietitian specializing in renal nutrition can help determine individualized sodium targets and develop a personalized meal plan tailored to specific dietary needs and health goals.

Identifying High-Sodium Foods:
Many processed and packaged foods are high in sodium, making them common culprits for excessive sodium intake. These include:
- Canned soups, broths, and sauces
- Processed meats such as deli meats, bacon, and sausage
- Snack foods like chips, pretzels, and crackers
- Condiments and seasonings such as soy sauce, ketchup, and seasoning blends
- Ready-to-eat meals, frozen dinners, and convenience foods
- Reading food labels and choosing low-sodium or sodium-free alternatives can help minimize sodium intake and support kidney health.

Strategies for Reducing Sodium Intake:
1. Cook at Home: Prepare meals from scratch using fresh, whole ingredients whenever possible. Cooking at home gives you greater control over the amount of salt added to your meals.
2. Use Herbs and Spices: Flavor your dishes with herbs, spices, citrus juices, vinegar, and other low-sodium seasonings to enhance taste without relying on salt.
3. Rinse and Drain: Rinse canned vegetables, beans, and other canned foods under running water to

remove excess sodium. Draining and rinsing can reduce sodium content by up to 40%.
4. Limit Processed Foods: Minimize consumption of processed and packaged foods, which are often high in sodium. Opt for fresh or frozen fruits and vegetables, lean meats, and low-sodium alternatives whenever possible.
5. Be Mindful When Dining Out: When eating out, request dishes to be prepared without added salt or sauces, and ask for dressings and condiments on the side. Choose grilled, steamed, or baked options over fried or heavily seasoned dishes.
6. Gradually Reduce Salt: Gradually decrease the amount of salt used in cooking and at the table to allow your taste buds to adjust to lower sodium levels. Experiment with herbs, spices, and other flavor enhancers to enhance the taste of your meals.
7. Monitor Food Labels: Read nutrition labels carefully and choose products labeled as "low sodium," "sodium-free," or "no added salt." Pay attention to serving sizes and sodium content per serving to make informed choices.
8. Stay Hydrated: Drinking an adequate amount of water can help flush out excess sodium from the body and maintain hydration, supporting kidney function and overall health.

Monitoring Sodium Intake and Blood Pressure:
1. Keep track of your daily sodium intake using a food diary or mobile app to ensure compliance with recommended guidelines. Regularly monitor blood pressure levels at home and report any significant changes to your healthcare provider.

2. Collaborate with a registered dietitian specializing in renal nutrition to review your dietary habits, identify sources of hidden sodium, and make adjustments as needed to optimize sodium intake and blood pressure control.

Achieving Balance in Potassium and Phosphorus Management

Maintaining optimal levels of potassium and phosphorus is crucial for individuals with kidney disease, as imbalances in these electrolytes can contribute to complications such as cardiovascular disease, bone disorders, and worsening kidney function. Achieving balance in potassium and phosphorus intake requires careful dietary management and close monitoring under the guidance of a healthcare provider or registered dietitian specializing in renal nutrition. Here's a detailed exploration of strategies to effectively manage potassium and phosphorus levels for kidney health:

Understanding Potassium and Phosphorus in Kidney Disease:
1. Potassium: Potassium is an essential mineral that plays a vital role in muscle function, nerve transmission, and fluid balance. However, individuals with kidney disease may experience difficulty regulating potassium levels, leading to hyperkalemia (high potassium levels) or hypokalemia (low potassium levels).
2. Phosphorus: Phosphorus is another important mineral involved in bone health, energy metabolism, and cellular function. Elevated phosphorus levels, known as hyperphosphatemia,

can occur in kidney disease due to decreased kidney function, leading to mineral and bone disorders (renal osteodystrophy) and cardiovascular complications.

Potassium Management:
1. Monitor Potassium Intake: Track your daily potassium intake and aim to maintain potassium levels within the recommended range. Work with a healthcare provider or renal dietitian to determine your individual potassium goals based on kidney function, medications, and other factors.
2. Choose Low-Potassium Foods: Include more low-potassium foods in your diet, such as apples, berries, cabbage, cauliflower, green beans, and rice. Limit high-potassium foods such as bananas, oranges, potatoes, tomatoes, spinach, and avocados, and consume them in moderation.
3. Cooking Methods: Certain cooking methods can help reduce potassium content in foods. Boiling, leaching, and soaking vegetables in water before cooking can help lower their potassium content. Drain and discard the soaking water to remove excess potassium.
4. Portion Control: Pay attention to portion sizes when consuming high-potassium foods. Eating smaller portions can help limit potassium intake while still enjoying a varied and nutritious diet.
5. Pharmacological Management: In some cases, medications such as potassium binders may be prescribed to help lower potassium levels in individuals with hyperkalemia. These medications bind to potassium in the gut, preventing its absorption into the bloodstream.

Phosphorus Management:
1. Limit Phosphorus-Rich Foods: Reduce consumption of phosphorus-rich foods such as dairy products, processed meats, nuts, seeds, and certain grains. Choose lower-phosphorus alternatives and opt for fresh, unprocessed foods whenever possible.
2. Read Food Labels: Check nutrition labels for phosphorus content and choose products labeled as "low phosphorus" or "phosphorus-free." Avoid additives such as phosphates and phosphoric acid commonly found in processed and packaged foods.
3. Calcium-Phosphorus Balance: Maintain a balance between calcium and phosphorus intake to prevent mineral imbalances and bone disorders. Consume adequate amounts of calcium-rich foods such as dairy products, fortified plant-based milks, and leafy green vegetables to help bind excess phosphorus in the gut and prevent its absorption.
4. Limit Phosphorus Additives: Minimize intake of processed foods containing phosphate additives, which are commonly found in baked goods, processed meats, and carbonated beverages. These additives can contribute to phosphorus overload and worsen kidney disease progression.
5. Phosphate Binders: In advanced stages of kidney disease, phosphate binders may be prescribed to help reduce phosphorus absorption from food. These medications bind to dietary phosphorus in the gut, preventing its absorption into the bloodstream and reducing circulating phosphorus levels.

Individualized Meal Planning:
1. Work with a registered dietitian specializing in renal nutrition to develop a personalized meal plan that balances potassium and phosphorus intake while meeting individual dietary needs, preferences, and health goals. A renal dietitian can provide guidance on portion control, food choices, cooking methods, and dining out while managing kidney disease.
2. Regularly monitor potassium and phosphorus levels through blood tests and adjust your dietary plan as needed in collaboration with your healthcare team. Tracking dietary changes and their impact on kidney function, electrolyte levels, and other relevant health markers is essential for optimizing kidney health and overall well-being.

Understanding Protein Consumption's Impact on Kidney Functions

Protein is an essential macronutrient that plays a vital role in various physiological functions, including muscle repair, immune function, hormone synthesis, and enzyme activity. However, in the context of kidney disease, managing protein consumption is a critical aspect of renal health. Understanding the impact of protein intake on kidney functions is essential for individuals with kidney disease to make informed dietary choices and optimize their overall well-being. Here's a detailed exploration of how protein consumption affects kidney functions:

Normal Kidney Function and Protein Metabolism:
1. In individuals with healthy kidneys, dietary protein is broken down into amino acids, the building blocks of proteins, during digestion. These amino acids are then absorbed into the bloodstream and utilized by the body for various physiological processes.
2. The kidneys play a crucial role in filtering waste products and excess substances from the bloodstream, including urea, a byproduct of protein metabolism. Urea is excreted from the body through urine, helping to maintain proper nitrogen balance and prevent toxic buildup in the bloodstream.

Impact of Protein on Kidney Function in Healthy Individuals:
1. In individuals with normal kidney function, moderate protein intake is generally well-tolerated and does not adversely affect kidney health. The kidneys efficiently excrete excess urea and other waste products, maintaining normal kidney function even with varying levels of protein intake.
2. High-protein diets, such as those commonly followed by athletes or bodybuilders, may temporarily increase the kidneys' workload due to the higher nitrogen load from increased protein metabolism. However, this increase in workload is typically well-managed by healthy kidneys and does not lead to long-term kidney damage in the absence of underlying kidney disease.

Protein Consumption and Kidney Disease:
1. In individuals with kidney disease, particularly those with reduced kidney function (e.g., chronic kidney disease), excessive protein intake can pose challenges to kidney health. The kidneys may struggle to efficiently filter and excrete the waste products generated from increased protein metabolism, leading to accumulation of urea and other nitrogenous waste products in the bloodstream.
2. High protein intake can exacerbate proteinuria (the presence of protein in the urine) and glomerular damage, further compromising kidney function over time. It can also contribute to metabolic acidosis, electrolyte imbalances, and progression of kidney disease.

Balancing Protein Intake in Kidney Disease:
1. The optimal level of protein intake for individuals with kidney disease depends on various factors, including the stage of kidney disease, degree of kidney function impairment, presence of proteinuria, nutritional status, and overall health status.
2. In general, individuals with kidney disease are advised to consume moderate amounts of high-quality protein while monitoring kidney function closely. High-quality protein sources include lean meats, poultry, fish, eggs, dairy products, and plant-based proteins like beans, lentils, tofu, and nuts.

3. Depending on individual needs, healthcare providers may recommend reducing protein intake to mitigate the risk of further kidney damage, particularly in advanced stages of kidney disease. However, overly restrictive protein intake should be avoided to prevent malnutrition and muscle wasting.
4. Working with a registered dietitian specializing in renal nutrition is crucial for developing a personalized meal plan that balances protein intake with other nutritional requirements while supporting kidney health and overall well-being.

Monitoring and Adjusting Protein Consumption:
1. Regular monitoring of kidney function, including serum creatinine levels, glomerular filtration rate (GFR), and urine protein excretion, is essential for assessing the impact of protein consumption on kidney health.
2. Healthcare providers may recommend adjusting protein intake based on changes in kidney function, nutritional status, and other health factors. Close communication with the healthcare team and adherence to dietary recommendations are essential for optimizing kidney health and slowing the progression of kidney disease.

Hydration and Fluid Control Essentials

Maintaining proper hydration and fluid balance is essential for supporting kidney health and optimizing renal function. Adequate hydration ensures efficient kidney filtration, electrolyte balance, waste removal, and overall cellular function. However, for individuals with kidney disease, managing fluid intake becomes a critical aspect of renal care, as impaired kidney function can lead to fluid retention, electrolyte imbalances, and other complications. Here's a comprehensive exploration of the essentials of hydration and fluid control for kidney health:

Importance of Hydration:
- Adequate hydration is vital for kidney health, as it helps support optimal blood flow to the kidneys, facilitates the excretion of waste products and toxins, and maintains proper electrolyte balance. Hydration also helps prevent urinary tract infections and kidney stone formation by promoting urine dilution and flushing out harmful substances from the urinary tract.
- Proper hydration supports overall well-being by promoting digestion, circulation, temperature regulation, joint lubrication, and cognitive function. Dehydration, on the other hand, can lead to fatigue, dizziness, headache, constipation, and impaired physical and cognitive performance.

Hydration Recommendations:
- The recommended daily fluid intake varies depending on factors such as age, gender, body weight, activity level, climate, and health status. In general, most adults are advised to consume about 8-10 cups (64-80 ounces) of fluids per day, which can include water, herbal teas, broth-based soups, and hydrating fruits and vegetables.
- Individuals with kidney disease may need to adjust their fluid intake based on their kidney function, urine output, fluid restrictions, and other medical considerations. Those on dialysis or with advanced kidney disease may require stricter fluid restrictions to avoid fluid overload and electrolyte imbalances.

Monitoring Hydration Status:
- Monitoring hydration status is essential for individuals with kidney disease to ensure adequate fluid intake without risking fluid overload or dehydration. Pay attention to thirst cues, urine output, urine color, and other signs of hydration status.
- Dark yellow or amber-colored urine may indicate dehydration, while pale yellow or straw-colored urine is a sign of adequate hydration. However, certain medications, vitamins, and medical conditions can affect urine color, so it's essential to consider other factors as well.
- Regular monitoring of body weight, blood pressure, and laboratory parameters such as serum electrolytes and blood urea nitrogen (BUN) levels can provide additional insights into hydration status and fluid balance.

Fluid Control in Kidney Disease:
- Individuals with kidney disease, especially those with reduced kidney function or fluid retention (edema), may need to restrict their fluid intake to prevent complications such as fluid overload, hypertension, pulmonary edema, and electrolyte imbalances.
- Work with a healthcare provider or renal dietitian to determine your individual fluid goals and develop a personalized fluid management plan tailored to your specific needs, preferences, and health status. Adjust fluid intake based on urine output, thirst, and medical recommendations.

Hydration Strategies for Kidney Health:
- Drink fluids evenly throughout the day rather than consuming large amounts at once to avoid overwhelming the kidneys and minimize fluctuations in fluid balance.
- Choose hydrating beverages such as water, herbal teas, diluted fruit juices, and electrolyte-replenishing drinks over sugary sodas, caffeinated beverages, and alcohol, which can contribute to dehydration and electrolyte imbalances.
- Monitor sodium intake and avoid excessive salt consumption, as sodium can lead to fluid retention and exacerbate hypertension in individuals with kidney disease.

- Be mindful of fluid-containing foods such as soups, stews, fruits, vegetables, and dairy products, which can contribute to overall fluid intake. Adjust portion sizes and choose low-sodium options when incorporating fluid-rich foods into your diet.

Treatment of Fluid Overload:
- In cases of fluid overload or severe fluid retention, healthcare providers may prescribe diuretic medications (water pills) to help increase urine output and reduce fluid accumulation in the body. Follow medication instructions carefully and report any adverse effects or concerns to your healthcare team.
- In advanced stages of kidney disease, individuals may require hemodialysis or peritoneal dialysis to remove excess fluid and waste products from the bloodstream when the kidneys are no longer able to perform these functions adequately.

Hydration During Exercise and Illness:
- Maintain adequate hydration during physical activity, as sweating can lead to fluid loss and dehydration. Drink water or electrolyte-replenishing beverages before, during, and after exercise to stay hydrated and replace lost fluids and electrolytes.
- During illness, such as vomiting, diarrhea, fever, or infection, fluid losses can increase, leading to dehydration and electrolyte imbalances. Drink small, frequent sips of clear fluids, oral rehydration solutions, or electrolyte drinks to replenish fluids and prevent dehydration.

Individualized Approach to Hydration:
- Every individual's fluid needs and tolerance may vary based on factors such as kidney function, medical history, medications, dietary habits, and lifestyle. Work closely with your healthcare team to develop a personalized hydration plan that meets your specific needs while supporting kidney health and overall well-being.
- Monitor changes in hydration status, kidney function, and overall health, and adjust fluid intake as needed in collaboration with your healthcare provider. Be proactive in addressing any concerns or questions related to hydration and fluid management to optimize kidney health and quality of life.

Creating Your Kidney-Friendly Kitchen

Transforming your kitchen into a kidney-friendly space is an essential step in managing kidney disease and supporting optimal renal health. By stocking your kitchen with wholesome ingredients, implementing renal-friendly cooking techniques, and making thoughtful choices about kitchen tools and equipment, you can create an environment that promotes nutritious eating while minimizing the risk of exacerbating kidney-related complications. Here's a detailed guide to creating your kidney-friendly kitchen:

Stocking Kidney-Friendly Ingredients:

Fill your pantry, refrigerator, and freezer with kidney-friendly ingredients that support renal health. Choose fresh, whole foods whenever possible and opt for low-sodium, low-phosphorus, and low-potassium options to meet dietary restrictions associated with kidney disease. Essential kidney-friendly pantry staples include:
1. Whole grains such as brown rice, quinoa, and whole wheat pasta
2. Lean proteins like skinless poultry, fish, tofu, and legumes
3. Fresh fruits and vegetables with lower potassium content, such as apples, berries, cucumbers, and green beans
4. Low-phosphorus dairy alternatives like almond milk or rice milk
5. Herbs, spices, and flavorings for enhancing taste without relying on salt
6. Read food labels carefully to identify hidden sources of sodium, phosphorus, and potassium in packaged foods, sauces, condiments, and

seasonings. Choose products labeled as "low sodium," "no added salt," "low phosphorus," or "no phosphorus additives" whenever possible.

Implementing Renal-Friendly Cooking Techniques:
Modify cooking methods to reduce sodium, phosphorus, and potassium content in meals while maximizing flavor and nutritional value. Consider the following renal-friendly cooking techniques:
1. Boiling and leaching vegetables to reduce potassium content
2. Using herbs, spices, citrus juices, and vinegar to season dishes instead of salt
3. Grilling, baking, broiling, or roasting proteins instead of frying or breading
4. Incorporating cooking liquids such as low-sodium broths, wine, or citrus juices to add moisture and flavor to dishes
5. Draining and rinsing canned beans, vegetables, and fish to reduce sodium and phosphorus content
6. Avoiding high-phosphorus additives such as phosphate-based baking powders and processed meats
7. Experiment with renal-friendly recipes and cooking techniques to discover delicious and nutritious meals that align with your dietary needs and preferences. Get creative in the kitchen while prioritizing renal health and flavor.

Choosing Kidney-Friendly Kitchen Tools and Equipment:
Select kitchen tools and equipment that facilitate kidney-friendly cooking and meal preparation. Invest in the following essentials:

1. Non-stick cookware to reduce the need for added fats and oils during cooking
2. Sharp knives for easy and precise cutting of fruits, vegetables, and proteins
3. Cutting boards designated for specific food groups to prevent cross-contamination and foodborne illness
4. Food processor or blender for pureeing fruits, vegetables, and legumes to create smooth textures
5. Slow cooker or pressure cooker for convenient and hands-off meal preparation with minimal added sodium or fat
6. Measuring cups and spoons for portion control and accurate ingredient measurements
7. Regularly maintain and clean your kitchen tools and equipment to ensure food safety and hygiene. Proper cleaning and storage practices help prevent bacterial contamination and foodborne illnesses.

Organizing Your Kitchen for Efficiency and Accessibility:
Arrange your kitchen space for efficiency and accessibility to streamline meal preparation and cooking. Consider the following organizational tips:
1. Store kidney-friendly ingredients and cooking utensils in easily accessible areas, such as lower cabinets and drawers, to minimize reaching and bending.
2. Group similar items together, such as grains, proteins, fruits, and vegetables, to facilitate meal planning and ingredient retrieval.
3. Label containers and storage bins to identify kidney-friendly ingredients and leftovers easily.

4. Keep countertops clear and clutter-free to provide ample workspace for meal preparation and cooking.
5. Utilize vertical storage solutions, such as shelves, racks, and hooks, to maximize storage space and keep kitchen essentials within reach.

Maintaining a Kidney-Friendly Environment:
1. Create a supportive environment that promotes kidney-friendly eating habits and healthy lifestyle choices. Encourage family members or household members to participate in meal planning, grocery shopping, and cooking to foster a sense of community and shared responsibility.
2. Educate yourself and your loved ones about kidney disease, dietary restrictions, and the importance of renal health. Share resources, recipes, and meal ideas to inspire healthy eating and empower others to make informed choices about their diet and lifestyle.
3. Stay connected with healthcare providers, dietitians, and support groups specializing in renal nutrition to receive personalized guidance, resources, and support on your journey to kidney health.

Smart Meal Planning Tips

Meal planning is a cornerstone of kidney health management, enabling individuals with kidney disease to make informed dietary choices, adhere to nutritional guidelines, and maintain optimal renal function. By strategically planning meals and snacks, you can ensure a balanced intake of nutrients while minimizing the risk of exacerbating kidney-related complications. Here are detailed meal planning tips to support kidney health effectively:

Understand Dietary Restrictions:
- Before embarking on meal planning, it's crucial to understand your specific dietary restrictions and nutritional requirements based on your kidney function, stage of kidney disease, comorbidities, medications, and other relevant factors.
- Consult with a registered dietitian specializing in renal nutrition to receive personalized guidance and recommendations tailored to your individual needs and health goals.

Focus on Balanced Nutrition:
- Prioritize balanced meals that include a variety of nutrient-dense foods from all food groups, including fruits, vegetables, whole grains, lean proteins, and healthy fats.
- Aim to incorporate a combination of macronutrients (carbohydrates, proteins, and fats) and micronutrients (vitamins and minerals) into your meals to support overall health and well-being.

Monitor Portion Sizes:
- Be mindful of portion sizes to prevent overeating and ensure appropriate calorie intake. Use measuring cups, spoons, or visual cues to estimate portion sizes and avoid excessive calorie consumption.

- Pay attention to serving sizes recommended for individuals with kidney disease, particularly for foods high in potassium, phosphorus, and sodium.

Include High-Quality Proteins:
- Incorporate lean sources of protein into your meals, such as skinless poultry, fish, tofu, eggs, and legumes. These protein sources are lower in saturated fat and phosphorus, making them ideal choices for kidney health.
- Adjust protein intake based on your individual needs, stage of kidney disease, and dietary restrictions. Consult with your healthcare provider or dietitian to determine the appropriate amount of protein for your diet.

Emphasize Plant-Based Foods:
- Include a variety of fruits and vegetables in your meals to provide essential vitamins, minerals, and antioxidants while keeping potassium and phosphorus levels in check.
- Opt for lower-potassium fruits and vegetables, such as apples, berries, cabbage, carrots, and green beans, and consider cooking methods that reduce potassium content, such as boiling or leaching.

Limit Sodium Intake:
- Reduce sodium intake by choosing low-sodium or sodium-free alternatives to processed and packaged foods. Use herbs, spices, lemon juice, vinegar, and other flavorings to enhance the taste of meals without adding extra salt.

- Read food labels carefully and choose products labeled as "low sodium," "no added salt," or "sodium-free." Aim to consume less than 2,300 milligrams of sodium per day, or even less if advised by your healthcare provider.

Manage Potassium and Phosphorus Levels:
- Monitor potassium and phosphorus intake by choosing foods lower in these minerals and limiting high-potassium and high-phosphorus foods. Work with your dietitian to develop a personalized meal plan that balances these electrolytes while meeting nutritional needs.
- Choose low-potassium fruits and vegetables, limit intake of high-phosphorus foods such as dairy products and processed meats, and consider using phosphate binders as prescribed by your healthcare provider.

Plan Ahead and Prep Meals:
- Set aside time each week for meal planning and preparation to streamline the cooking process and ensure healthy eating habits. Create a weekly meal plan, make a grocery list, and prepare ingredients in advance to save time and effort during busy weekdays.
- Batch cook staple ingredients such as grains, beans, and proteins to have ready-to-eat components on hand for quick and convenient meals throughout the week.

Be Flexible and Creative:
- Stay flexible with your meal planning approach and be open to trying new recipes, ingredients, and

cooking methods. Get creative in the kitchen by experimenting with different flavors, textures, and cuisines to keep meals interesting and enjoyable.
- Modify recipes to suit your dietary needs and preferences, substituting ingredients as needed to accommodate renal restrictions while maintaining flavor and nutrition.

Listen to Your Body:
Pay attention to how your body responds to different foods and meals, and adjust your meal plan accordingly. Keep a food diary to track your intake, symptoms, and overall well-being, and share this information with your healthcare team or dietitian for personalized guidance.

Part 3: Staying Active for Healthy Kidney

Harnessing the Benefits of Regular Exercise for Kidney Health

Regular exercise is a cornerstone of a healthy lifestyle and offers numerous benefits for kidney health. Engaging in physical activity can help individuals with kidney disease improve cardiovascular fitness, manage blood pressure, maintain muscle strength, enhance mood, and support overall well-being. By incorporating regular exercise into their routine, individuals with kidney disease can optimize renal function, reduce the risk of complications, and improve their quality of life. Here's a detailed exploration of the benefits of regular exercise for kidney health:

Improving Cardiovascular Fitness:
- Regular exercise, including aerobic activities such as walking, jogging, cycling, swimming, or dancing, can improve cardiovascular fitness and endurance. These activities help strengthen the heart muscle, enhance circulation, and increase oxygen delivery to tissues throughout the body, including the kidneys.
- Improved cardiovascular fitness can reduce the risk of cardiovascular complications associated with kidney disease, such as hypertension, heart disease, and stroke. By promoting heart health, exercise supports overall renal function and reduces the burden on the kidneys.

Managing Blood Pressure:
- Exercise plays a crucial role in managing blood pressure, a key risk factor for kidney disease progression and cardiovascular events. Regular physical activity helps lower blood pressure by improving blood vessel function, reducing arterial stiffness, and promoting vasodilation.
- Aerobic exercise, in particular, has been shown to lower both systolic and diastolic blood pressure in individuals with hypertension and chronic kidney disease. By lowering blood pressure, exercise helps protect the kidneys from damage and reduces the risk of complications such as kidney failure and cardiovascular events.

Maintaining Muscle Strength and Function:
- Muscle wasting and weakness are common complications of kidney disease, especially in individuals on dialysis or with advanced kidney failure. Regular exercise, including resistance training or strength-based exercises, can help preserve muscle mass, improve muscle strength, and enhance physical function.
- Strength training exercises, such as lifting weights, using resistance bands, or performing bodyweight exercises, stimulate muscle growth, increase bone density, and improve functional capacity. Strong muscles support overall mobility, balance, and independence, contributing to better quality of life for individuals with kidney disease.

Enhancing Mood and Mental Well-Being:
- Exercise has been shown to have positive effects on mental health and well-being, including reducing symptoms of depression, anxiety, and stress. Regular physical activity stimulates the release of endorphins, neurotransmitters that promote feelings of happiness and relaxation.
- Individuals with kidney disease may experience emotional challenges, including depression, anxiety, and social isolation, due to the burden of managing a chronic illness. Engaging in regular exercise can help alleviate these symptoms, improve mood, and enhance overall mental well-being.

Supporting Weight Management and Metabolic Health:
- Exercise plays a crucial role in supporting weight management and metabolic health, which are important considerations for individuals with kidney disease. Regular physical activity helps regulate metabolism, increase energy expenditure, and promote fat loss while preserving lean muscle mass.
- Maintaining a healthy weight and body composition is essential for managing risk factors such as obesity, insulin resistance, and dyslipidemia, which can contribute to kidney disease progression and cardiovascular complications.

Promoting Kidney Function and Longevity:
- While exercise cannot reverse kidney damage or cure kidney disease, it can help slow the progression of kidney disease and improve overall kidney health. Regular physical activity promotes optimal blood flow to the kidneys, enhances oxygenation of renal tissues, and supports waste removal through increased urine output.
- Studies have shown that individuals who engage in regular exercise have better renal outcomes and a lower risk of kidney disease progression compared to sedentary individuals. By promoting kidney function and reducing the risk of complications, exercise supports longevity and improves overall quality of life for individuals with kidney disease.

Practical Considerations for Exercise in Kidney Disease:
- Before starting an exercise program, individuals with kidney disease should consult with their healthcare provider or nephrologist to assess their overall health status, identify any potential contraindications or precautions, and receive personalized exercise recommendations.
- When beginning an exercise program, start slowly and gradually increase the duration, intensity, and frequency of activity over time. Aim for at least 150 minutes of moderate-intensity aerobic exercise or 75 minutes of vigorous-intensity aerobic exercise per week, as recommended by guidelines for adults.
- Incorporate a variety of activities into your routine, including aerobic exercise, strength training, flexibility exercises, and balance training, to

promote overall fitness and prevent injury. Choose activities that you enjoy and can sustain long-term to maintain motivation and adherence.
- Stay hydrated before, during, and after exercise, especially in individuals with kidney disease who may have fluid restrictions or electrolyte imbalances. Monitor symptoms such as fatigue, dizziness, shortness of breath, or chest pain during exercise and adjust intensity or duration as needed.
- Be mindful of potential complications or risks associated with exercise in kidney disease, such as electrolyte imbalances, fluid shifts, or musculoskeletal injuries. Work with a qualified fitness professional or physical therapist with experience in kidney disease management to develop a safe and effective exercise program tailored to your individual needs and goals.

Safe and Effective Workouts Tailored for Women with Kidney Diseases

Exercise is an integral component of managing kidney disease and promoting overall health and well-being in women. However, it's crucial for individuals with kidney diseases to engage in safe and effective workouts that accommodate their unique needs, medical considerations, and fitness levels. Tailoring exercise regimens to address the specific challenges and limitations associated with kidney diseases can help women maximize the benefits of physical activity while minimizing the risk of complications. Here's a detailed exploration of safe and effective workouts tailored for women with kidney diseases:

Consultation with Healthcare Provider:
- Before starting any exercise program, women with kidney diseases should consult with their healthcare provider, preferably a nephrologist or primary care physician familiar with their medical history and kidney function.
- Healthcare providers can assess the individual's overall health status, kidney function, cardiovascular risk factors, medications, and potential contraindications to exercise. They can provide personalized recommendations and guidance on safe exercise modalities based on the individual's specific needs and medical considerations.

Individualized Exercise Prescription:
- Exercise programs for women with kidney diseases should be tailored to their unique needs, preferences, fitness levels, and medical conditions. An individualized exercise prescription takes into account factors such as kidney function, cardiovascular health, musculoskeletal status, mobility limitations, and any comorbidities.
- The exercise prescription may include recommendations for aerobic exercise, strength training, flexibility exercises, balance training, and functional movements, depending on the individual's goals and capabilities.

Cardiovascular Exercise:
- Cardiovascular exercise, also known as aerobic exercise, is essential for improving cardiovascular fitness, managing blood pressure, and supporting overall health in women with kidney diseases. Safe and effective cardiovascular exercises for women with kidney diseases include:
- Walking: A low-impact, accessible activity that can be performed indoors or outdoors at a moderate intensity.
- Cycling: Stationary cycling or outdoor biking can provide a cardiovascular workout while minimizing joint stress.
- Swimming or water aerobics: Water-based exercises are gentle on the joints and offer resistance for cardiovascular conditioning.
- Elliptical training or low-impact aerobics: Using elliptical machines or participating in low-impact aerobic classes can provide a cardiovascular workout without excessive joint strain.

Strength Training:
- Strength training, also known as resistance training, is beneficial for preserving muscle mass, improving muscular strength, and enhancing functional capacity in women with kidney diseases. Incorporating strength training exercises into the workout regimen can help maintain bone density, improve metabolic health, and support activities of daily living.
- Safe and effective strength training exercises for women with kidney diseases include:

- Bodyweight exercises: Squats, lunges, push-ups, and planks can be performed using body weight as resistance.
- Resistance band exercises: Using resistance bands provides adjustable resistance for various muscle groups without the need for heavy weights.
- Light dumbbell or kettlebell exercises: Using light weights under supervision can help improve muscular strength and endurance safely.
- Machines or equipment with adjustable resistance: Selecting machines or equipment that allow for controlled resistance adjustments can accommodate individual fitness levels and progressions.

Flexibility and Stretching:
- Flexibility exercises and stretching are essential components of an exercise program for women with kidney diseases. Stretching helps improve joint range of motion, reduce muscle tension, prevent injuries, and enhance overall flexibility and mobility.
- Incorporate gentle stretching exercises into the workout routine to target major muscle groups and improve flexibility. Focus on static stretching, holding each stretch for 15-30 seconds without bouncing, to gradually lengthen muscles and increase range of motion.
-
- Balance and Stability Training:
- Balance and stability training exercises are beneficial for improving balance, coordination, and proprioception in women with kidney

diseases. These exercises help reduce the risk of falls, enhance postural control, and promote functional independence.
- Incorporate balance exercises into the workout routine, such as standing on one leg, heel-to-toe walking, or using balance boards or stability balls to challenge balance and stability. Start with simple exercises and progress gradually as balance improves.

Hydration and Fluid Management:
- Women with kidney diseases should pay special attention to hydration and fluid management during exercise to prevent dehydration and electrolyte imbalances. Stay adequately hydrated before, during, and after exercise by drinking water or electrolyte-replenishing beverages as needed.
- Follow fluid intake recommendations provided by healthcare providers, especially for individuals with fluid restrictions or electrolyte imbalances. Monitor hydration status and adjust fluid intake based on individual needs, environmental conditions, and exercise intensity.

Monitoring Symptoms and Adjusting Exercise Intensity:
- Women with kidney diseases should listen to their bodies and pay attention to any signs or symptoms that may indicate exercise-related complications. Common symptoms to monitor during exercise include fatigue, dizziness, shortness of breath, chest pain, palpitations, and muscle cramps.
- If experiencing any discomfort or adverse symptoms during exercise, stop the activity immediately and seek medical attention if

necessary. Adjust exercise intensity, duration, or type as needed to ensure safety and minimize the risk of complications.

Regular Monitoring and Progression:
- Regular monitoring of exercise progress, kidney function, and overall health status is essential for women with kidney diseases. Track exercise frequency, duration, intensity, and perceived exertion to assess progress and identify areas for improvement.
- Work closely with healthcare providers, including nephrologists, physical therapists, and exercise professionals, to evaluate exercise tolerance, adjust exercise prescriptions, and monitor changes in kidney function over time.

Lifestyle Integration and Sustainability:
- Integrating exercise into daily life and establishing sustainable habits is key to long-term success in managing kidney diseases. Encourage women with kidney diseases to find activities they enjoy, set realistic goals, and prioritize consistency and adherence.
- Incorporate physical activity into daily routines, such as taking the stairs instead of the elevator, walking or cycling for transportation, gardening, or participating in recreational activities with friends and family. Making exercise a fun and enjoyable part of life can enhance motivation and adherence.

Incorporating Movement into Daily Life

Leading a sedentary lifestyle can have detrimental effects on kidney health and overall well-being. Incorporating movement into daily life is essential for individuals, particularly those with kidney diseases, to improve cardiovascular fitness, maintain muscle strength, support weight management, and enhance overall health. By making small, intentional changes to daily routines, individuals can increase physical activity levels, reduce sedentary behavior, and reap the benefits of a more active lifestyle. Here's a detailed exploration of strategies for incorporating movement into daily life:

Set Realistic Goals:
- Start by setting achievable goals for increasing daily physical activity. Begin with small, manageable changes and gradually increase the duration, intensity, and frequency of movement over time.
- Aim for at least 150 minutes of moderate-intensity aerobic activity or 75 minutes of vigorous-intensity aerobic activity per week, as recommended by guidelines for adults. Break down activity into shorter sessions throughout the day if needed.

Find Opportunities to Move:
- Look for opportunities to incorporate movement into daily activities, such as household chores, errands, work tasks, and recreational pursuits. Every bit of movement counts, whether it's taking the stairs instead of the elevator, parking farther

away from destinations, or standing up and stretching during breaks.
- Be creative and find activities that you enjoy and can integrate seamlessly into your daily routine. Experiment with different types of movement, such as walking, cycling, swimming, dancing, gardening, or playing with pets or children.

Prioritize Daily Walks:
- Walking is one of the simplest and most accessible forms of physical activity that can be incorporated into daily life. Aim to take short walks throughout the day, whether it's during breaks at work, after meals, or in the evening with family or friends.
- Set a goal to accumulate steps gradually, starting with a manageable target and increasing step count over time. Use a pedometer, smartphone app, or fitness tracker to track daily steps and stay motivated to meet activity goals.

Active Transportation:
- Consider incorporating active transportation into your daily commute or errands by walking, cycling, or using public transportation. Walking or cycling to work, school, or nearby destinations not only provides physical activity but also reduces carbon emissions and promotes environmental sustainability.
- Plan walking or cycling routes that are safe, convenient, and enjoyable, and explore scenic trails, parks, or green spaces in your community. Invite family members, friends, or coworkers to join you for a walk or bike ride to make it a social activity.

Take Active Breaks:
- Break up long periods of sitting or sedentary behavior with short active breaks throughout the day. Set reminders to stand up, stretch, and move around every hour, especially if you have a desk-bound job or spend extended periods sitting.
- Incorporate simple exercises or stretches into your routine to improve circulation, relieve muscle tension, and promote mobility. Perform leg lifts, arm circles, shoulder rolls, or seated yoga poses to increase blood flow and energy levels.

Household Chores and Gardening:
- Household chores and gardening offer opportunities to engage in physical activity while accomplishing necessary tasks around the home. Vacuuming, sweeping, mopping, dusting, and gardening activities such as planting, weeding, and watering can provide a full-body workout.
- Dedicate time each week to tackle household chores and gardening tasks, and view them as opportunities to move your body, burn calories, and maintain a clean and organized living space.

Stay Active with Hobbies and Recreation:
- Incorporate physical activity into hobbies and recreational pursuits that you enjoy. Whether it's dancing, swimming, playing sports, practicing yoga, or participating in outdoor activities like hiking or kayaking, find activities that bring you joy and fulfillment.

- Schedule regular time for hobbies and recreational activities, and prioritize self-care by engaging in activities that promote physical, mental, and emotional well-being. Invite friends or family members to join you for social support and motivation.

Make Movement Fun and Enjoyable:
- Choose activities that you find enjoyable, stimulating, and rewarding to maintain motivation and adherence to a more active lifestyle. Experiment with different types of movement and discover activities that resonate with your interests, preferences, and abilities.
- Incorporate variety into your routine to prevent boredom and keep exercise sessions fresh and engaging. Mix and match different activities, try new classes or workouts, and explore outdoor environments to stay inspired and motivated.

Listen to Your Body and Rest as Needed:
- Pay attention to your body's signals and adjust your activity level accordingly. Be mindful of fatigue, discomfort, or pain, and take breaks or rest days as needed to prevent overexertion or injury.
- Balance physical activity with rest and recovery to allow your body to repair and recharge. Incorporate relaxation techniques such as deep breathing, meditation, or gentle stretching to promote stress reduction and enhance recovery.

Stay Consistent and Celebrate Progress:
- Stay committed to incorporating movement into daily life by establishing consistent habits and

routines. Celebrate small victories and milestones along the way, whether it's reaching a step goal, improving endurance, or mastering a new activity.
- Keep a journal or log of your physical activity to track progress, set new goals, and reflect on accomplishments. Celebrate your commitment to health and well-being and acknowledge the positive impact that movement has on your overall quality of life.

Exploring the Vital Role of Sleep in Kidney Function

Sleep plays a crucial role in overall health and well-being, and its impact on kidney function is significant. Adequate and restorative sleep is essential for maintaining optimal renal health, supporting metabolic processes, regulating blood pressure, and promoting overall physiological balance. Conversely, disruptions in sleep patterns or sleep disorders can have adverse effects on kidney function and contribute to the development or progression of kidney diseases. Here's a detailed exploration of the vital role of sleep in kidney function:

Regulation of Renal Processes:
- Sleep is a period of physiological rest and recovery during which the body undergoes essential repair and restoration processes. During sleep, the kidneys play a crucial role in maintaining fluid balance, electrolyte homeostasis, and waste excretion through urine production.
- The kidneys continue to filter blood and regulate blood pressure, electrolyte levels, and acid-base balance during sleep. Adequate sleep allows for

optimal kidney function and efficient removal of metabolic waste products, toxins, and excess fluids from the body.

Blood Pressure Regulation:
- Sleep plays a key role in regulating blood pressure, which is closely linked to kidney function. During sleep, blood pressure typically decreases, allowing the cardiovascular system to rest and recover. This nighttime dip in blood pressure, known as nocturnal dipping, is essential for cardiovascular health and renal perfusion.
- Disruptions in sleep patterns, such as sleep deprivation or sleep disorders like sleep apnea, can impair nocturnal dipping and lead to elevated blood pressure levels throughout the day. Chronic hypertension is a significant risk factor for kidney diseases and can contribute to kidney damage over time.

Inflammation and Immune Function:
- Adequate sleep is essential for supporting immune function and reducing inflammation in the body. During sleep, the immune system releases cytokines and other signaling molecules that help regulate immune responses, promote tissue repair, and combat infections.
- Chronic sleep deprivation or poor sleep quality can dysregulate immune function and promote systemic inflammation, which may contribute to the development or progression of kidney diseases. Inflammatory processes play a role in the pathogenesis of various kidney disorders, including glomerulonephritis, diabetic nephropathy, and chronic kidney disease.

Metabolic Regulation:
- Sleep influences metabolic processes such as glucose metabolism, insulin sensitivity, and lipid regulation, all of which can impact kidney health. Adequate sleep is essential for maintaining metabolic homeostasis and preventing metabolic imbalances that can contribute to kidney dysfunction.
- Sleep disturbances, such as short sleep duration or sleep fragmentation, have been associated with metabolic disorders such as obesity, insulin resistance, and dyslipidemia, which are risk factors for kidney diseases. Improving sleep quality and duration may help mitigate these metabolic risks and support renal health.

Stress and Hormonal Balance:
- Sleep plays a role in regulating stress hormones and hormonal balance, which can impact kidney function and overall health. Chronic stress and dysregulation of stress hormones such as cortisol can contribute to hypertension, inflammation, and oxidative stress, all of which are detrimental to kidney health.
- Adequate sleep helps modulate the hypothalamic-pituitary-adrenal (HPA) axis and promotes hormonal balance, which is essential for managing stress responses and maintaining physiological equilibrium. Chronic sleep deprivation or poor sleep quality can disrupt HPA axis function and

exacerbate stress-related health conditions, including kidney diseases.

Management of Sleep Disorders in Kidney Disease:
- Individuals with kidney diseases, especially those on dialysis or with advanced chronic kidney disease (CKD), are at increased risk of sleep disorders such as obstructive sleep apnea (OSA), restless legs syndrome (RLS), and insomnia. These sleep disorders can negatively impact sleep quality, exacerbate symptoms of kidney disease, and contribute to poor health outcomes.
- Management of sleep disorders in individuals with kidney disease requires a multidisciplinary approach involving nephrologists, sleep specialists, and other healthcare providers. Treatment modalities may include lifestyle modifications, continuous positive airway pressure (CPAP) therapy for OSA, medications, behavioral therapies, and addressing underlying medical conditions contributing to sleep disturbances.

Promoting Healthy Sleep Habits:
- Adopting healthy sleep habits, also known as sleep hygiene practices, is essential for optimizing sleep quality and supporting kidney health. Strategies for promoting healthy sleep habits include:
- Establishing a regular sleep schedule: Go to bed and wake up at the same time each day, even on weekends, to regulate your body's internal clock.
- Creating a relaxing bedtime routine: Wind down before bed with calming activities such as reading,

listening to soothing music, or taking a warm bath to signal to your body that it's time to sleep.
- Creating a sleep-conducive environment: Keep your bedroom dark, quiet, and cool, and invest in a comfortable mattress and pillows to promote restful sleep.
- Limiting exposure to screens and stimulating activities before bed: Avoid electronic devices, bright lights, and stimulating activities that can interfere with melatonin production and disrupt sleep onset.
- Avoiding caffeine, alcohol, and heavy meals close to bedtime: Limit consumption of stimulants and large meals in the evening, as they can interfere with sleep quality and digestion.

Seeking Professional Help When Needed:
If you're experiencing persistent sleep disturbances or symptoms of sleep disorders, such as snoring, daytime fatigue, or difficulty falling or staying asleep, consult with a healthcare provider or sleep specialist for evaluation and management. Addressing sleep disorders promptly can improve sleep quality, enhance overall health, and support kidney function.

PART 4: HEALTHY AND DELICIOUS RECIPES

Breakfast Recipes

Vegetable Omelette

Ingredients:
2 eggs
1/4 cup diced bell peppers
1/4 cup diced onions
1/4 cup diced tomatoes
1 tablespoon olive oil
Salt and pepper to taste

Preparation:
Heat olive oil in a non-stick skillet over medium heat.
Sauté bell peppers, onions, and tomatoes until tender.
Beat eggs in a bowl and pour over the sautéed vegetables.
Cook until the omelette is set, then fold in half.
Season with salt and pepper to taste.
Nutritional Information (per serving):
Sodium: 200 mg
Potassium: 270 mg
Phosphorus: 150 mg
Protein: 12 g
Calories: 180

Greek Yogurt Parfait

Ingredients:
1/2 cup plain Greek yogurt
1/4 cup fresh berries (such as strawberries, blueberries, or raspberries)
2 tablespoons chopped nuts (almonds or walnuts)
1 tablespoon honey (optional)

Preparation:
Layer Greek yogurt, berries, and nuts in a serving glass or bowl.
Drizzle with honey if desired.
Serve chilled.
Nutritional Information (per serving):
Sodium: 50 mg
Potassium: 200 mg
Phosphorus: 100 mg
Protein: 10 g
Calories: 150

Spinach and Mushroom Frittata

Ingredients:
4 eggs
1 cup chopped spinach
1/2 cup sliced mushrooms
1/4 cup diced onions
1 tablespoon olive oil
Salt and pepper to taste

Preparation:
Preheat oven to 350°F (175°C).
Heat olive oil in an oven-safe skillet over medium heat.
Sauté spinach, mushrooms, and onions until tender.
In a bowl, beat eggs and season with salt and pepper.
Pour eggs over the sautéed vegetables in the skillet.
Transfer skillet to the oven and bake for 15-20 minutes until the frittata is set.
Slice and serve.
Nutritional Information (per serving):
Sodium: 220 mg
Potassium: 310 mg
Phosphorus: 160 mg
Protein: 14 g
Calories: 200

Quinoa Breakfast Bowl

Ingredients:
1/2 cup cooked quinoa
1/4 cup sliced strawberries
1/4 cup diced mango
2 tablespoons chopped almonds
1 tablespoon honey (optional)

Preparation:
Cook quinoa according to package instructions.
In a bowl, combine cooked quinoa, strawberries, mango, and almonds.
Drizzle with honey if desired.
Serve warm or chilled.
Nutritional Information (per serving):

Sodium: 5 mg
Potassium: 180 mg
Phosphorus: 120 mg
Protein: 6 g
Calories: 180

Avocado Toast with Poached Egg

Ingredients:
1 slice whole grain bread
1/2 ripe avocado, mashed
1 poached egg
Salt and pepper to taste

Preparation:
Toast the whole grain bread until golden brown.
Spread mashed avocado evenly on the toasted bread.
Top with a poached egg.
Season with salt and pepper to taste.
Nutritional Information (per serving):
Sodium: 200 mg
Potassium: 370 mg
Phosphorus: 150 mg
Protein: 10 g
Calories: 220

Banana Walnut Smoothie

Ingredients:
1 ripe banana
1/4 cup chopped walnuts
1/2 cup plain Greek yogurt
1/2 cup almond milk (unsweetened)

1 teaspoon honey (optional)

Preparation:
Place all ingredients in a blender.
Blend until smooth and creamy.
Add more almond milk if needed to reach desired consistency.
Sweeten with honey if desired.
Nutritional Information (per serving):
Sodium: 50 mg
Potassium: 380 mg
Phosphorus: 120 mg
Protein: 10 g
Calories: 250

Cottage Cheese and Fruit Bowl

Ingredients:
1/2 cup low-fat cottage cheese
1/4 cup diced pineapple
1/4 cup sliced peaches
2 tablespoons sliced almonds

Preparation:
Spoon cottage cheese into a serving bowl.
Top with diced pineapple, sliced peaches, and sliced almonds.
Serve chilled.
Nutritional Information (per serving):
Sodium: 220 mg
Potassium: 260 mg
Phosphorus: 150 mg
Protein: 14 g

Calories: 200

Whole Grain Pancakes with Berries

Ingredients:
1/2 cup whole wheat flour
1/4 cup oat flour
1 teaspoon baking powder
1/4 teaspoon cinnamon
1/2 cup almond milk (unsweetened)
1 egg
1/2 cup mixed berries (blueberries, strawberries, raspberries)
1 tablespoon maple syrup (optional)

Preparation:
In a mixing bowl, combine whole wheat flour, oat flour, baking powder, and cinnamon.
Add almond milk and egg to the dry ingredients and mix until smooth.
Heat a non-stick skillet over medium heat and lightly coat with cooking spray.
Pour batter onto the skillet to form pancakes.
Cook until bubbles form on the surface, then flip and cook until golden brown.
Serve topped with mixed berries and drizzled with maple syrup if desired.
Nutritional Information (per serving):
Sodium: 150 mg
Potassium: 220 mg
Phosphorus: 180 mg
Protein: 8 g

Calories: 220

Egg and Veggie Breakfast Burrito

Ingredients:
1 whole grain tortilla
2 eggs, scrambled
1/4 cup diced bell peppers
1/4 cup diced onions
1/4 cup diced tomatoes
1 tablespoon salsa
Salt and pepper to taste

Preparation:
Heat a non-stick skillet over medium heat.
Add diced bell peppers, onions, and tomatoes to the skillet and sauté until tender.
Add scrambled eggs to the skillet and cook until set.
Season with salt and pepper to taste.
Warm the tortilla in the skillet or microwave.
Spoon the egg and veggie mixture onto the tortilla, top with salsa, and fold into a burrito.
Nutritional Information (per serving):
Sodium: 250 mg
Potassium: 270 mg
Phosphorus: 170 mg
Protein: 12 g
Calories: 230

Mediterranean Breakfast Bowl

Ingredients:
1/2 cup cooked quinoa
1/4 cup cherry tomatoes, halved
1/4 cup cucumber, diced
2 tablespoons crumbled feta cheese
1 tablespoon chopped fresh parsley
1 tablespoon lemon juice
1 tablespoon olive oil
Salt and pepper to taste

Preparation:
In a bowl, combine cooked quinoa, cherry tomatoes, cucumber, feta cheese, and parsley.
Drizzle with lemon juice and olive oil.
Season with salt and pepper to taste.
Toss gently to combine.
Nutritional Information (per serving):
Sodium: 180 mg
Potassium: 230 mg
Phosphorus: 180 mg
Protein: 8 g
Calories: 210

Blueberry Almond Chia Pudding

Ingredients:
1/4 cup chia seeds
1 cup almond milk (unsweetened)
1/4 cup fresh blueberries
2 tablespoons sliced almonds
1 teaspoon honey (optional)

Preparation:
In a jar or bowl, mix chia seeds and almond milk.
Stir well to combine and let sit for at least 30 minutes or overnight in the refrigerator until thickened.
Before serving, top with fresh blueberries and sliced almonds.
Drizzle with honey if desired.
Nutritional Information (per serving):
Sodium: 80 mg
Potassium: 140 mg
Phosphorus: 100 mg
Protein: 6 g
Calories: 170

Turkey and Veggie Breakfast Wrap

Ingredients:
1 whole grain tortilla
2 slices turkey breast
1/4 cup baby spinach leaves
1/4 cup diced tomatoes
1 tablespoon hummus
Salt and pepper to taste

Preparation:
Spread hummus evenly on the whole grain tortilla.
Layer turkey breast slices, baby spinach leaves, and diced tomatoes on top of the hummus.
Season with salt and pepper to taste.
Roll up the tortilla into a wrap and slice in half if desired.
Nutritional Information (per serving):
Sodium: 250 mg
Potassium: 280 mg

Phosphorus: 200 mg
Protein: 10 g
Calories: 200

Sweet Potato and Black Bean Breakfast Hash

Ingredients:
1 small sweet potato, diced
1/4 cup canned black beans, rinsed and drained
1/4 cup diced bell peppers
1/4 cup diced onions
1 tablespoon olive oil
1/2 teaspoon smoked paprika
Salt and pepper to taste

Preparation:
Heat olive oil in a skillet over medium heat.
Add diced sweet potato to the skillet and cook until tender and golden brown.
Add diced bell peppers and onions to the skillet and sauté until softened.
Stir in black beans, smoked paprika, salt, and pepper.
Cook for an additional 2-3 minutes until heated through.
Serve hot as a breakfast hash.
Nutritional Information (per serving):
Sodium: 220 mg
Potassium: 280 mg
Phosphorus: 180 mg
Protein: 8 g
Calories: 220

Apple Cinnamon Overnight Oats

Ingredients:
1/2 cup rolled oats
1/2 cup almond milk (unsweetened)
1/4 cup plain Greek yogurt
1/2 apple, diced
1 tablespoon chopped walnuts
1/2 teaspoon ground cinnamon
1 teaspoon honey (optional)

Preparation:
In a jar or bowl, combine rolled oats, almond milk, Greek yogurt, diced apple, chopped walnuts, and ground cinnamon.
Stir well to combine.
Cover and refrigerate overnight or for at least 4 hours.
Before serving, drizzle with honey if desired.
Nutritional Information (per serving):
Sodium: 70 mg
Potassium: 210 mg
Phosphorus: 150 mg
Protein: 8 g
Calories: 210

Lunch Recipes

Grilled Lemon Herb Chicken Salad

Ingredients:
4 oz grilled chicken breast, sliced
2 cups mixed greens
1/4 cup cherry tomatoes, halved
1/4 cucumber, sliced
1 tablespoon chopped fresh herbs (such as parsley, basil, or cilantro)
1 tablespoon lemon juice
1 tablespoon olive oil
Salt and pepper to taste

Preparation:
In a bowl, toss mixed greens, cherry tomatoes, cucumber, and fresh herbs.
Arrange grilled chicken slices on top of the salad.
Drizzle with lemon juice and olive oil.
Season with salt and pepper to taste.
Nutritional Information (per serving):
Sodium: 150 mg
Potassium: 300 mg
Phosphorus: 200 mg
Protein: 25 g
Calories: 250

Quinoa and Black Bean Stuffed Bell Peppers

Ingredients:
2 large bell peppers, halved and seeded
1 cup cooked quinoa
1/2 cup canned black beans, rinsed and drained
1/4 cup diced tomatoes
1/4 cup diced onions
1/4 cup shredded low-fat cheese
1 teaspoon olive oil
1/2 teaspoon ground cumin
Salt and pepper to taste

Preparation:
Preheat the oven to 375°F (190°C).
In a skillet, heat olive oil over medium heat.
Sauté diced onions until translucent.
Add cooked quinoa, black beans, diced tomatoes, ground cumin, salt, and pepper. Cook until heated through.
Stuff bell pepper halves with the quinoa and black bean mixture.
Sprinkle shredded cheese on top of each stuffed pepper.
Bake in the preheated oven for 20-25 minutes until peppers are tender and cheese is melted.
Nutritional Information (per serving):
Sodium: 200 mg
Potassium: 380 mg
Phosphorus: 250 mg
Protein: 12 g
Calories: 280

Salmon and Asparagus Quiche

Ingredients:
1 pre-made whole grain pie crust
6 oz cooked salmon, flaked
1 cup chopped asparagus
1/4 cup diced onions
1/2 cup low-fat milk
4 eggs
1/4 cup shredded low-fat cheese
Salt and pepper to taste

Preparation:
Preheat the oven to 375°F (190°C).
Place pie crust in a pie dish and set aside.
In a skillet, sauté chopped asparagus and diced onions until tender.
Spread cooked salmon, asparagus, and onions evenly in the pie crust.
In a bowl, whisk together eggs, low-fat milk, salt, and pepper.
Pour egg mixture over the salmon and asparagus in the pie crust.
Sprinkle shredded cheese on top.
Bake in the preheated oven for 30-35 minutes until the quiche is set and the crust is golden brown.
Nutritional Information (per serving):
Sodium: 240 mg
Potassium: 360 mg
Phosphorus: 250 mg
Protein: 20 g
Calories: 320

Vegetarian Lentil Soup

Ingredients:
1 cup dry lentils, rinsed and drained
4 cups low-sodium vegetable broth
1/2 cup diced carrots
1/2 cup diced celery
1/4 cup diced onions
2 cloves garlic, minced
1 teaspoon olive oil
1 teaspoon dried thyme
Salt and pepper to taste

Preparation:
In a large pot, heat olive oil over medium heat.
Sauté diced onions and minced garlic until fragrant.
Add diced carrots and celery to the pot and cook until slightly softened.
Stir in dry lentils, dried thyme, salt, and pepper.
Pour low-sodium vegetable broth into the pot and bring to a boil.
Reduce heat to low, cover, and simmer for 25-30 minutes until lentils are tender.
Adjust seasoning with salt and pepper as needed.
Nutritional Information (per serving):
Sodium: 120 mg
Potassium: 400 mg
Phosphorus: 180 mg
Protein: 15 g
Calories: 220

Tuna Salad Lettuce Wraps

Ingredients:
1 can (5 oz) water-packed tuna, drained
2 tablespoons plain Greek yogurt
1 tablespoon Dijon mustard
1/4 cup diced celery
1/4 cup diced red bell pepper
1 tablespoon chopped fresh parsley
Salt and pepper to taste
4 large lettuce leaves (such as butter or romaine)

Preparation:
In a bowl, mix drained tuna, Greek yogurt, Dijon mustard, diced celery, diced red bell pepper, chopped parsley, salt, and pepper.
Spoon tuna salad onto lettuce leaves.
Roll up the lettuce leaves to form wraps.
Serve immediately.
Nutritional Information (per serving):
Sodium: 220 mg
Potassium: 350 mg
Phosphorus: 200 mg
Protein: 20 g
Calories: 180

Mushroom and Spinach Whole Grain Pasta

Ingredients:
2 cups whole grain pasta (such as penne or fusilli)
1 cup sliced mushrooms
2 cups baby spinach leaves
2 cloves garlic, minced
2 tablespoons olive oil
2 tablespoons grated Parmesan cheese
Salt and pepper to taste

Preparation:
Cook whole grain pasta according to package instructions. Drain and set aside.
In a skillet, heat olive oil over medium heat.
Sauté minced garlic until fragrant.
Add sliced mushrooms to the skillet and cook until golden brown.
Stir in baby spinach leaves and cooked pasta.
Cook until spinach wilts and pasta is heated through.
Season with salt and pepper to taste.
Sprinkle grated Parmesan cheese on top before serving.
Nutritional Information (per serving):
Sodium: 180 mg
Potassium: 320 mg
Phosphorus: 200 mg
Protein: 10 g
Calories: 240

Chickpea and Avocado Salad

Ingredients:
1 can (15 oz) chickpeas, rinsed and drained
1 ripe avocado, diced
1/4 cup diced red onion
1/4 cup chopped fresh cilantro
1 tablespoon lime juice
1 tablespoon olive oil
Salt and pepper to taste

Preparation:
In a large bowl, combine chickpeas, diced avocado, diced red onion, and chopped cilantro.
Drizzle with lime juice and olive oil.
Season with salt and pepper to taste.
Toss gently to combine.
Nutritional Information (per serving):
Sodium: 220 mg
Potassium: 390 mg
Phosphorus: 180 mg
Protein: 10 g
Calories: 230

Turkey and Veggie Wrap

Ingredients:
1 whole grain tortilla
2 slices turkey breast
1/4 cup shredded lettuce
1/4 cup sliced cucumber
1/4 cup sliced bell peppers
1 tablespoon hummus

Salt and pepper to taste

Preparation:
Spread hummus evenly on the whole grain tortilla.
Layer turkey breast slices, shredded lettuce, sliced cucumber, and sliced bell peppers on top of the hummus.
Season with salt and pepper to taste.
Roll up the tortilla into a wrap and slice in half if desired.
Nutritional Information (per serving):
Sodium: 250 mg
Potassium: 280 mg
Phosphorus: 200 mg
Protein: 10 g
Calories: 200

Sesame Ginger Tofu Stir-Fry

Ingredients:
1 block (14 oz) extra-firm tofu, cubed
2 cups mixed vegetables (such as bell peppers, broccoli, and snap peas)
2 cloves garlic, minced
2 tablespoons low-sodium soy sauce
1 tablespoon sesame oil
1 tablespoon rice vinegar
1 tablespoon honey (optional)
1 tablespoon sesame seeds
Salt and pepper to taste

Preparation:
Heat sesame oil in a large skillet or wok over medium heat.

Add minced garlic and cubed tofu to the skillet and cook until tofu is golden brown on all sides.
Stir in mixed vegetables and cook until tender-crisp.
In a small bowl, whisk together low-sodium soy sauce, rice vinegar, and honey.
Pour the sauce over the tofu and vegetable mixture in the skillet.
Toss to coat evenly and cook for an additional 2-3 minutes.
Sprinkle sesame seeds on top before serving.
Nutritional Information (per serving):
Sodium: 300 mg
Potassium: 430 mg
Phosphorus: 250 mg
Protein: 15 g
Calories: 280

Caprese Quinoa Salad

Ingredients:
1 cup cooked quinoa
1 cup cherry tomatoes, halved
1/2 cup fresh mozzarella balls (bocconcini), halved
1/4 cup chopped fresh basil
1 tablespoon balsamic vinegar
1 tablespoon olive oil
Salt and pepper to taste

Preparation:
In a large bowl, combine cooked quinoa, cherry tomatoes, fresh mozzarella balls, and chopped basil.
Drizzle with balsamic vinegar and olive oil.
Season with salt and pepper to taste.

Toss gently to combine.
Nutritional Information (per serving):
Sodium: 220 mg
Potassium: 320 mg
Phosphorus: 180 mg
Protein: 10 g
Calories: 240

Vegetable and Bean Chili

Ingredients:
1 can (15 oz) low-sodium kidney beans, rinsed and drained
1 can (15 oz) low-sodium black beans, rinsed and drained
1 can (15 oz) diced tomatoes
1 cup chopped bell peppers
1 cup diced zucchini
1/2 cup diced onions
2 cloves garlic, minced
1 tablespoon olive oil
1 tablespoon chili powder
1 teaspoon ground cumin
Salt and pepper to taste

Preparation:
In a large pot, heat olive oil over medium heat.
Sauté diced onions and minced garlic until fragrant.
Add chopped bell peppers and diced zucchini to the pot and cook until slightly softened.
Stir in low-sodium kidney beans, low-sodium black beans, diced tomatoes, chili powder, ground cumin, salt, and pepper.

Bring the chili to a simmer and cook for 20-25 minutes until vegetables are tender and flavors are blended.
Adjust seasoning with salt and pepper as needed.
Nutritional Information (per serving):
Sodium: 200 mg
Potassium: 450 mg
Phosphorus: 250 mg
Protein: 12 g
Calories: 270

Eggplant and Tomato Pasta

Ingredients:
2 cups whole grain pasta (such as penne or spaghetti)
1 small eggplant, diced
1 cup cherry tomatoes, halved
2 cloves garlic, minced
2 tablespoons olive oil
1 tablespoon balsamic vinegar
1 tablespoon chopped fresh basil
Salt and pepper to taste

Preparation:
Cook whole grain pasta according to package instructions. Drain and set aside.
In a large skillet, heat olive oil over medium heat.
Sauté minced garlic until fragrant.
Add diced eggplant to the skillet and cook until tender.
Stir in halved cherry tomatoes and cooked pasta.
Drizzle with balsamic vinegar and sprinkle with chopped fresh basil.
Season with salt and pepper to taste.
Nutritional Information (per serving):

Sodium: 180 mg
Potassium: 320 mg
Phosphorus: 200 mg
Protein: 8 g
Calories: 230

Turkey and Bean Chili

Ingredients:
1 lb ground turkey
1 can (15 oz) low-sodium kidney beans, rinsed and drained
1 can (15 oz) diced tomatoes
1 cup chopped bell peppers
1 cup diced onions
2 cloves garlic, minced
2 tablespoons olive oil
1 tablespoon chili powder
1 teaspoon ground cumin
Salt and pepper to taste

Preparation:
In a large pot, heat olive oil over medium heat.
Sauté diced onions and minced garlic until fragrant.
Add ground turkey to the pot and cook until browned.
Stir in chopped bell peppers, low-sodium kidney beans, diced tomatoes, chili powder, ground cumin, salt, and pepper.
Bring the chili to a simmer and cook for 20-25 minutes until flavors are blended.
Adjust seasoning with salt and pepper as needed.
Nutritional Information (per serving):
Sodium: 220 mg

Potassium: 450 mg
Phosphorus: 300 mg
Protein: 20 g
Calories: 290

Mediterranean Chickpea Salad

Ingredients:
1 can (15 oz) chickpeas, rinsed and drained
1 cup cherry tomatoes, halved
1/2 cup diced cucumber
1/4 cup diced red onion
1/4 cup chopped fresh parsley
2 tablespoons crumbled feta cheese
1 tablespoon olive oil
1 tablespoon lemon juice
Salt and pepper to taste

Preparation:
In a large bowl, combine chickpeas, cherry tomatoes, diced cucumber, diced red onion, chopped fresh parsley, and crumbled feta cheese.
Drizzle with olive oil and lemon juice.
Season with salt and pepper to taste.
Toss gently to combine.
Nutritional Information (per serving):
Sodium: 230 mg
Potassium: 380 mg
Phosphorus: 200 mg
Protein: 10 g
Calories: 240

Dinner Recipes

Baked Lemon Herb Salmon

Ingredients:
4 oz salmon fillet
1 tablespoon fresh lemon juice
1 teaspoon olive oil
1 clove garlic, minced
1/2 teaspoon dried dill
Salt and pepper to taste

Preparation:
Preheat the oven to 375°F (190°C).
In a small bowl, mix together lemon juice, olive oil, minced garlic, dried dill, salt, and pepper.
Place the salmon fillet on a baking sheet lined with parchment paper.
Brush the lemon herb mixture evenly over the salmon.
Bake in the preheated oven for 12-15 minutes until the salmon is cooked through and flakes easily with a fork.
Nutritional Information (per serving):
Sodium: 180 mg
Potassium: 350 mg

Phosphorus: 250 mg
Protein: 25 g
Calories: 280

Vegetable Stir-Fry with Tofu

Ingredients:
1 block (14 oz) extra-firm tofu, cubed
2 cups mixed vegetables (such as bell peppers, broccoli, and carrots)
2 cloves garlic, minced
2 tablespoons low-sodium soy sauce
1 tablespoon sesame oil
1 tablespoon rice vinegar
1 tablespoon honey (optional)
Salt and pepper to taste

Preparation:
Heat sesame oil in a large skillet or wok over medium heat.
Add minced garlic and cubed tofu to the skillet and cook until tofu is golden brown on all sides.
Stir in mixed vegetables and cook until tender-crisp.
In a small bowl, whisk together low-sodium soy sauce, rice vinegar, and honey.
Pour the sauce over the tofu and vegetable mixture in the skillet.

Toss to coat evenly and cook for an additional 2-3 minutes.
Season with salt and pepper to taste.
Nutritional Information (per serving):
Sodium: 280 mg
Potassium: 420 mg
Phosphorus: 280 mg
Protein: 20 g
Calories: 290

Baked Chicken and Vegetable Casserole

Ingredients:
4 oz boneless, skinless chicken breast
1 cup diced potatoes
1 cup diced carrots
1 cup green beans, trimmed and halved
1/4 cup low-sodium chicken broth
1 tablespoon olive oil
1 teaspoon dried thyme
Salt and pepper to taste

Preparation:
Preheat the oven to 375°F (190°C).
Place diced potatoes, carrots, and green beans in a baking dish.
Drizzle with olive oil and sprinkle with dried thyme, salt, and pepper. Toss to coat evenly.
Place the chicken breast on top of the vegetables.
Pour low-sodium chicken broth over the chicken and vegetables.

Cover the baking dish with foil and bake in the preheated oven for 25-30 minutes.
Remove the foil and bake for an additional 10-15 minutes until the chicken is cooked through and vegetables are tender.
Nutritional Information (per serving):
Sodium: 200 mg
Potassium: 400 mg
Phosphorus: 250 mg
Protein: 25 g
Calories: 300

Turkey and Vegetable Quinoa Bowl

Ingredients:
1/2 cup cooked quinoa
4 oz ground turkey
1/2 cup mixed vegetables (such as bell peppers, zucchini, and mushrooms)
1/4 cup diced tomatoes
1 tablespoon olive oil
1/2 teaspoon ground cumin
Salt and pepper to taste

Preparation:
Heat olive oil in a skillet over medium heat.
Add ground turkey to the skillet and cook until browned.
Stir in mixed vegetables and diced tomatoes. Cook until vegetables are tender.
Sprinkle ground cumin, salt, and pepper over the turkey and vegetable mixture.

Serve the turkey and vegetable mixture over cooked quinoa.
Nutritional Information (per serving):
Sodium: 220 mg
Potassium: 350 mg
Phosphorus: 200 mg
Protein: 20 g
Calories: 270

Eggplant Parmesan

Ingredients:
1 medium eggplant, sliced into rounds
1/2 cup whole wheat breadcrumbs
1/4 cup grated Parmesan cheese
1 egg, beaten
1 cup marinara sauce (low-sodium)
1/2 cup shredded mozzarella cheese
1 tablespoon olive oil
Salt and pepper to taste

Preparation:
Preheat the oven to 375°F (190°C).
Dip eggplant slices in beaten egg, then coat with a mixture of whole wheat breadcrumbs, grated Parmesan cheese, salt, and pepper.

Place coated eggplant slices on a baking sheet lined with parchment paper.
Drizzle olive oil over the eggplant slices.
Bake in the preheated oven for 20-25 minutes until eggplant is tender and breadcrumbs are golden brown.
Remove from the oven and top each eggplant slice with marinara sauce and shredded mozzarella cheese.
Return to the oven and bake for an additional 5-7 minutes until the cheese is melted and bubbly.
Nutritional Information (per serving):
Sodium: 220 mg
Potassium: 320 mg
Phosphorus: 200 mg
Protein: 15 g
Calories: 280

Vegetarian Lentil Curry

Ingredients:
1 cup dry lentils, rinsed and drained
1 can (14 oz) diced tomatoes
1 cup diced potatoes
1 cup chopped carrots
1/2 cup diced onions
2 cloves garlic, minced
1 tablespoon curry powder
1 teaspoon ground cumin
1 teaspoon ground turmeric
1/4 teaspoon cayenne pepper (optional)
Salt and pepper to taste

Preparation:

In a large pot, combine dry lentils, diced tomatoes, diced potatoes, chopped carrots, diced onions, minced garlic, curry powder, ground cumin, ground turmeric, cayenne pepper (if using), salt, and pepper.

Add enough water to cover the ingredients by 1 inch.

Bring the mixture to a boil, then reduce heat to low, cover, and simmer for 25-30 minutes until lentils and vegetables are tender.

Adjust seasoning with salt and pepper as needed.

Nutritional Information (per serving):
Sodium: 180 mg
Potassium: 380 mg
Phosphorus: 200 mg
Protein: 15 g
Calories: 250

Grilled Chicken Caesar Salad

Ingredients:
4 oz grilled chicken breast, sliced
2 cups romaine lettuce, chopped
1/4 cup cherry tomatoes, halved
2 tablespoons grated Parmesan cheese
2 tablespoons Caesar dressing (low-sodium)
1 tablespoon whole wheat croutons
Salt and pepper to taste

Preparation:
In a large bowl, combine chopped romaine lettuce, cherry tomatoes, and grated Parmesan cheese.

Drizzle Caesar dressing over the salad and toss to coat evenly.
Transfer the salad to a serving plate and top with sliced grilled chicken breast.
Garnish with whole wheat croutons.
Season with salt and pepper to taste.
Nutritional Information (per serving):
Sodium: 220 mg
Potassium: 300 mg
Phosphorus: 200 mg
Protein: 25 g
Calories: 280

Turkey Meatball and Vegetable Skewers

Ingredients:
4 oz lean ground turkey
1/4 cup whole wheat breadcrumbs
1/4 cup grated Parmesan cheese
1/4 cup diced bell peppers
1/4 cup diced zucchini
1/4 cup diced red onion
1 tablespoon olive oil
Salt and pepper to taste
Wooden skewers, soaked in water

Preparation:
Preheat the grill or grill pan over medium heat.
In a bowl, mix together ground turkey, whole wheat breadcrumbs, grated Parmesan cheese, diced bell peppers, diced zucchini, diced red onion, salt, and pepper until well combined.
Form the mixture into small meatballs.

Thread the meatballs and diced vegetables onto the soaked wooden skewers, alternating between them.

Brush the skewers with olive oil and season with salt and pepper.

Grill the skewers for 10-12 minutes, turning occasionally, until the turkey meatballs are cooked through and the vegetables are tender.

Nutritional Information (per serving):

Sodium: 230 mg

Potassium: 320 mg

Phosphorus: 200 mg

Protein: 20 g

Calories: 270

Stuffed Bell Peppers with Quinoa and Black Beans

Ingredients:
2 large bell peppers, halved and seeded
1 cup cooked quinoa
1/2 cup canned black beans, rinsed and drained
1/4 cup diced tomatoes
1/4 cup diced onions
1/4 cup shredded low-fat cheese
1 teaspoon olive oil
1/2 teaspoon ground cumin
Salt and pepper to taste

Preparation:
Preheat oven to 375°F (190°C).
In a skillet, heat olive oil over medium heat.
Sauté diced onions until translucent.
Add cooked quinoa, black beans, diced tomatoes, ground cumin, salt, and pepper. Cook until heated through.
Stuff bell pepper halves with the quinoa and black bean mixture.
Sprinkle shredded cheese on top of each stuffed pepper.
Bake in the preheated oven for 20-25 minutes until peppers are tender and cheese is melted.
Nutritional Information (per serving):
Sodium: 200 mg
Potassium: 380 mg
Phosphorus: 250 mg
Protein: 12 g
Calories: 280

Mediterranean Grilled Vegetable Platter

Ingredients:
1 zucchini, sliced lengthwise
1 yellow squash, sliced lengthwise
1 eggplant, sliced into rounds
1 red bell pepper, seeded and quartered
1 yellow bell pepper, seeded and quartered
1 red onion, sliced into thick rings
2 tablespoons olive oil
1 tablespoon balsamic vinegar
1 teaspoon dried oregano
Salt and pepper to taste

Preparation:
Preheat the grill or grill pan over medium-high heat.
In a bowl, whisk together olive oil, balsamic vinegar, dried oregano, salt, and pepper.
Brush the sliced vegetables with the olive oil mixture.
Grill the vegetables for 3-4 minutes per side until tender and lightly charred.
Arrange the grilled vegetables on a platter and serve hot.
Nutritional Information (per serving):
Sodium: 160 mg
Potassium: 350 mg
Phosphorus: 150 mg
Protein: 5 g
Calories: 180

Sautéed Shrimp with Garlic and Spinach

Ingredients:
6 oz shrimp, peeled and deveined
2 cups fresh spinach leaves
2 cloves garlic, minced
1 tablespoon olive oil
1 tablespoon lemon juice
Salt and pepper to taste

Preparation:
Heat olive oil in a skillet over medium heat.
Add minced garlic and sauté until fragrant.
Add shrimp to the skillet and cook until pink and opaque, about 2-3 minutes per side.
Stir in fresh spinach leaves and cook until wilted.
Drizzle lemon juice over the shrimp and spinach.
Season with salt and pepper to taste.
Serve hot.
Nutritional Information (per serving):
Sodium: 220 mg
Potassium: 320 mg
Phosphorus: 200 mg
Protein: 20 g
Calories: 230

Teriyaki Tofu Stir-Fry

Ingredients:
1 block (14 oz) extra-firm tofu, cubed

2 cups mixed vegetables (such as bell peppers, broccoli, and snap peas)
2 cloves garlic, minced
2 tablespoons low-sodium soy sauce
1 tablespoon teriyaki sauce (low-sodium)
1 tablespoon sesame oil
Salt and pepper to taste

Preparation:
Heat sesame oil in a large skillet or wok over medium heat.
Add minced garlic and cubed tofu to the skillet and cook until tofu is golden brown on all sides.
Stir in mixed vegetables and cook until tender-crisp.
In a small bowl, whisk together low-sodium soy sauce and teriyaki sauce.
Pour the sauce over the tofu and vegetable mixture in the skillet.
Toss to coat evenly and cook for an additional 2-3 minutes.
Season with salt and pepper to taste.
Nutritional Information (per serving):
Sodium: 280 mg
Potassium: 420 mg
Phosphorus: 250 mg
Protein: 20 g
Calories: 290

Lemon Garlic Chicken with Roasted Vegetables

Ingredients:
4 oz chicken breast

1 cup mixed vegetables (such as carrots, Brussels sprouts, and cauliflower)
1 tablespoon olive oil
1 tablespoon fresh lemon juice
2 cloves garlic, minced
1 teaspoon dried thyme
Salt and pepper to taste

Preparation:
Preheat oven to 375°F (190°C).
In a bowl, whisk together olive oil, fresh lemon juice, minced garlic, dried thyme, salt, and pepper.
Place chicken breast and mixed vegetables on a baking sheet lined with parchment paper.
Brush the olive oil mixture over the chicken and vegetables.
Bake in the preheated oven for 20-25 minutes until the chicken is cooked through and vegetables are tender.
Nutritional Information (per serving):
Sodium: 180 mg
Potassium: 350 mg
Phosphorus: 250 mg
Protein: 25 g
Calories: 280

Salmon and Asparagus Foil Packets

Ingredients:
4 oz salmon fillet
1 cup asparagus spears
1/4 cup diced tomatoes
1 tablespoon olive oil
1 tablespoon fresh lemon juice

1 teaspoon minced garlic
Salt and pepper to taste

Preparation:
Preheat oven to 375°F (190°C).
Place a piece of aluminum foil on a baking sheet.
Arrange salmon fillet, asparagus spears, and diced tomatoes on the foil.
Drizzle with olive oil and fresh lemon juice.
Sprinkle minced garlic, salt, and pepper over the salmon and vegetables.
Fold the foil over the salmon and vegetables to create a packet, sealing the edges tightly.
Bake in the preheated oven for 15-20 minutes until salmon is cooked through and vegetables are tender.
Nutritional Information (per serving):
Sodium: 200 mg
Potassium: 370 mg
Phosphorus: 250 mg
Protein: 25 g
Calories: 290

Dessert Recipes

Berry Parfait

Ingredients:
1/2 cup low-fat Greek yogurt
1/4 cup mixed berries (such as strawberries, blueberries, and raspberries)
1 tablespoon honey (optional)
1 tablespoon crushed nuts (such as almonds or walnuts)

Preparation:
In a glass or bowl, layer low-fat Greek yogurt, mixed berries, and honey (if using) alternately.
Top with crushed nuts.
Serve chilled.
Nutritional Information (per serving):
Sodium: 50 mg
Potassium: 200 mg
Phosphorus: 100 mg
Protein: 10 g
Calories: 120

Frozen Banana Bites

Ingredients:
2 ripe bananas, peeled and sliced into rounds
1/4 cup melted dark chocolate (unsweetened)
2 tablespoons chopped nuts (such as peanuts or almonds)

Preparation:

Dip banana slices into melted dark chocolate, then place them on a parchment-lined baking sheet.
Sprinkle chopped nuts over the chocolate-coated banana slices.
Freeze for 1-2 hours until the chocolate is set.
Serve chilled.
Nutritional Information (per serving):
Sodium: 5 mg
Potassium: 200 mg
Phosphorus: 50 mg
Protein: 2 g
Calories: 90

Coconut Chia Pudding

Ingredients:
1/4 cup chia seeds
1 cup coconut milk (unsweetened)
1 tablespoon honey (optional)
1/4 teaspoon vanilla extract
1 tablespoon shredded coconut (unsweetened), for garnish

Preparation:
In a bowl, mix together chia seeds, coconut milk, honey (if using), and vanilla extract.
Cover and refrigerate for at least 2 hours or overnight until the mixture thickens.
Stir well before serving and garnish with shredded coconut.
Nutritional Information (per serving):
Sodium: 20 mg
Potassium: 150 mg
Phosphorus: 70 mg

Protein: 3 g
Calories: 120

Baked Apple with Cinnamon

Ingredients:
1 apple, cored and sliced
1 teaspoon cinnamon
1 tablespoon honey (optional)
1 tablespoon chopped nuts (such as pecans or almonds)

Preparation:
Preheat the oven to 375°F (190°C).
Place apple slices in a baking dish and sprinkle with cinnamon.
Drizzle with honey (if using) and sprinkle with chopped nuts.
Bake in the preheated oven for 15-20 minutes until apples are tender.
Serve warm.
Nutritional Information (per serving):
Sodium: 0 mg
Potassium: 150 mg
Phosphorus: 20 mg
Protein: 1 g
Calories: 80

Yogurt Bark with Berries

Ingredients:
1 cup low-fat Greek yogurt
1/4 cup mixed berries (such as strawberries, blueberries, and raspberries)

1 tablespoon honey (optional)

Preparation:
Line a baking sheet with parchment paper.
Spread low-fat Greek yogurt evenly on the parchment paper.
Sprinkle mixed berries over the yogurt and drizzle with honey (if using).
Freeze for 2-3 hours until firm.
Break into pieces and serve chilled.
Nutritional Information (per serving):
Sodium: 30 mg
Potassium: 150 mg
Phosphorus: 70 mg
Protein: 6 g
Calories: 100

Peanut Butter Banana Smoothie

Ingredients:
1 ripe banana
2 tablespoons natural peanut butter
1 cup unsweetened almond milk
1/2 teaspoon vanilla extract
Ice cubes (optional)

Preparation:
In a blender, combine ripe banana, natural peanut butter, unsweetened almond milk, and vanilla extract.
Blend until smooth.
Add ice cubes if desired and blend again until creamy.
Pour into glasses and serve immediately.

Nutritional Information (per serving):
Sodium: 110 mg
Potassium: 350 mg
Phosphorus: 100 mg
Protein: 6 g
Calories: 180

Frozen Yogurt Bark with Mango

Ingredients:
1 cup low-fat Greek yogurt
1/2 cup diced mango
1 tablespoon honey (optional)

Preparation:
Line a baking sheet with parchment paper.
Spread low-fat Greek yogurt evenly on the parchment paper.
Sprinkle diced mango over the yogurt and drizzle with honey (if using).
Freeze for 2-3 hours until firm.
Break into pieces and serve chilled.
Nutritional Information (per serving):
Sodium: 30 mg
Potassium: 200 mg
Phosphorus: 70 mg
Protein: 6 g
Calories: 110

Blueberry Oatmeal Cookies

Ingredients:
1 cup rolled oats

1/2 cup whole wheat flour
1/4 cup mashed banana
1/4 cup unsweetened applesauce
1/4 cup blueberries (fresh or frozen)
1 tablespoon honey (optional)
1/2 teaspoon vanilla extract

Preparation:
Preheat the oven to 350°F (175°C) and line a baking sheet with parchment paper.
In a bowl, combine rolled oats, whole wheat flour, mashed banana, unsweetened applesauce, blueberries, honey (if using), and vanilla extract. Mix well to form a dough.
Scoop spoonfuls of dough onto the prepared baking sheet, flattening them slightly with a fork.
Bake for 12-15 minutes until golden brown.
Allow to cool before serving.
Nutritional Information (per serving):
Sodium: 40 mg
Potassium: 100 mg
Phosphorus: 60 mg
Protein: 2 g
Calories: 80

Chocolate Avocado Mousse

Ingredients:
1 ripe avocado, peeled and pitted
2 tablespoons unsweetened cocoa powder
2 tablespoons honey (or maple syrup)
1/2 teaspoon vanilla extract
Pinch of salt
Optional toppings: sliced strawberries or raspberries

Preparation:
In a blender or food processor, combine avocado, cocoa powder, honey (or maple syrup), vanilla extract, and a pinch of salt.
Blend until smooth and creamy.
Transfer the mousse to serving bowls and refrigerate for at least 30 minutes to chill.
Serve with sliced strawberries or raspberries if desired.
Nutritional Information (per serving):
Sodium: 5 mg
Potassium: 200 mg
Phosphorus: 60 mg
Protein: 2 g
Calories: 120

Cinnamon Baked Apples

Ingredients:
2 apples, cored and halved
1 tablespoon melted butter (or coconut oil)
1 tablespoon honey (or maple syrup)
1/2 teaspoon ground cinnamon
1/4 teaspoon ground nutmeg
Optional toppings: Greek yogurt or chopped nuts

Preparation:
Preheat the oven to 375°F (190°C) and line a baking dish with parchment paper.
Place apple halves in the baking dish.
In a small bowl, mix melted butter (or coconut oil), honey (or maple syrup), ground cinnamon, and ground nutmeg.
Drizzle the mixture over the apple halves.

Bake for 20-25 minutes until apples are tender.
Serve warm with a dollop of Greek yogurt or chopped nuts if desired.
Nutritional Information (per serving):
Sodium: 5 mg
Potassium: 100 mg
Phosphorus: 20 mg
Protein: 0 g
Calories: 70

Peach Sorbet

Ingredients:
2 ripe peaches, peeled and sliced
1 tablespoon honey (or maple syrup)
1 tablespoon lemon juice
1/4 cup water

Preparation:
Place peach slices in a blender or food processor.
Add honey (or maple syrup), lemon juice, and water.
Blend until smooth.
Pour the mixture into a shallow dish and freeze for 2-3 hours, stirring every 30 minutes until firm.
Serve scoops of peach sorbet in bowls.
Nutritional Information (per serving):
Sodium: 0 mg
Potassium: 150 mg
Phosphorus: 20 mg
Protein: 1 g
Calories: 60

Chia Seed Pudding with Strawberries

Ingredients:
1/4 cup chia seeds
1 cup unsweetened almond milk
1 tablespoon honey (or maple syrup)
1/2 teaspoon vanilla extract
1/2 cup sliced strawberries
Preparation:
In a bowl, mix together chia seeds, almond milk, honey (or maple syrup), and vanilla extract.
Cover and refrigerate for at least 2 hours or overnight until the mixture thickens.
Stir well before serving and top with sliced strawberries.
Nutritional Information (per serving):
Sodium: 20 mg
Potassium: 100 mg
Phosphorus: 60 mg
Protein: 3 g
Calories: 90

Watermelon Mint Salad

Ingredients:
2 cups diced watermelon
1 tablespoon chopped fresh mint leaves
1 tablespoon lime juice
1 teaspoon honey (optional)

Preparation:
In a bowl, combine diced watermelon, chopped fresh mint leaves, lime juice, and honey (if using).

Toss gently to coat the watermelon evenly with the mint and lime mixture.
Serve chilled.
Nutritional Information (per serving):
Sodium: 0 mg
Potassium: 200 mg
Phosphorus: 10 mg
Protein: 1 g
Calories: 50

Mixed Berry Smoothie Bowl

Ingredients:
1/2 cup mixed berries (such as strawberries, blueberries, and raspberries)
1/2 banana
1/2 cup low-fat Greek yogurt
1/4 cup unsweetened almond milk
Optional toppings: sliced banana, granola, shredded coconut

Preparation:
In a blender, combine mixed berries, banana, low-fat Greek yogurt, and unsweetened almond milk.
Blend until smooth.
Pour the smoothie into a bowl and add toppings as desired.
Nutritional Information (per serving):
Sodium: 50 mg
Potassium: 200 mg
Phosphorus: 70 mg
Protein: 6 g
Calories: 120

Pineapple Coconut Ice Pops

Ingredients:
2 cups diced pineapple
1/2 cup coconut water
1 tablespoon honey (or maple syrup)
1/4 cup shredded coconut (unsweetened)

Preparation:
In a blender, combine diced pineapple, coconut water, and honey (or maple syrup).
Blend until smooth.
Stir in shredded coconut.
Pour the mixture into ice pop molds and insert sticks.
Freeze for at least 4 hours until firm.
Nutritional Information (per serving):
Sodium: 20 mg
Potassium: 200 mg
Phosphorus: 50 mg
Protein: 1 g
Calories: 70

Snacks Recipes

Cucumber Hummus Bites

Ingredients:
1 cucumber, sliced into rounds
1/4 cup hummus (low-sodium)

1 tablespoon chopped parsley
Salt and pepper to taste

Preparation:
Spread a small amount of hummus on each cucumber round.
Sprinkle chopped parsley over the hummus.
Season with salt and pepper to taste.
Nutritional Information (per serving):
Sodium: 60 mg
Potassium: 150 mg
Phosphorus: 50 mg
Protein: 2 g
Calories: 30

Greek Yogurt with Berries and Almonds

Ingredients:
1/2 cup low-fat Greek yogurt
1/4 cup mixed berries (such as blueberries and strawberries)
1 tablespoon sliced almonds
1 teaspoon honey (optional)

Preparation:
In a bowl, layer low-fat Greek yogurt, mixed berries, and sliced almonds.
Drizzle with honey (if using) for added sweetness.
Nutritional Information (per serving):
Sodium: 40 mg
Potassium: 200 mg
Phosphorus: 60 mg
Protein: 8 g

Calories: 100

Rice Cake with Avocado and Tomato

Ingredients:
1 rice cake (low-sodium)
1/4 avocado, mashed
1 small tomato, sliced
Salt and pepper to taste

Preparation:
Spread mashed avocado onto the rice cake.
Top with sliced tomato.
Season with salt and pepper to taste.
Nutritional Information (per serving):
Sodium: 30 mg
Potassium: 150 mg
Phosphorus: 50 mg
Protein: 2 g
Calories: 70

Edamame Salad

Ingredients:
1 cup cooked edamame (shelled)
1/4 cup diced cucumber
1/4 cup diced bell pepper
1 tablespoon chopped cilantro
1 tablespoon rice vinegar (low-sodium)
1 teaspoon sesame oil
Salt and pepper to taste

Preparation:
In a bowl, combine cooked edamame, diced cucumber, diced bell pepper, and chopped cilantro.
Drizzle with rice vinegar and sesame oil.
Season with salt and pepper to taste.
Nutritional Information (per serving):
Sodium: 10 mg
Potassium: 200 mg
Phosphorus: 50 mg
Protein: 8 g
Calories: 90

Caprese Skewers

Ingredients:
Cherry tomatoes
Fresh mozzarella balls
Fresh basil leaves
Balsamic glaze (optional)
Wooden skewers

Preparation:
Thread cherry tomatoes, fresh mozzarella balls, and fresh basil leaves onto wooden skewers.
Drizzle with balsamic glaze if desired.
Nutritional Information (per serving):
Sodium: 80 mg
Potassium: 150 mg
Phosphorus: 100 mg
Protein: 5 g
Calories: 70

Turkey and Cheese Roll-Ups

Ingredients:
2 slices low-sodium turkey breast
2 slices low-fat cheese
1 tablespoon mustard (low-sodium)

Preparation:
Spread mustard on each slice of turkey breast.
Place a slice of cheese on top of the turkey slice.
Roll up tightly and secure with toothpicks if needed.
Nutritional Information (per serving):
Sodium: 120 mg
Potassium: 90 mg
Phosphorus: 120 mg
Protein: 15 g
Calories: 120

Fruit Salad with Mint

Ingredients:
1 cup mixed fruits (such as pineapple, mango, and kiwi), diced
1 tablespoon chopped fresh mint leaves
1 teaspoon honey (optional)

Preparation:
In a bowl, combine diced mixed fruits and chopped fresh mint leaves.
Drizzle with honey (if using) for added sweetness.
Nutritional Information (per serving):
Sodium: 0 mg
Potassium: 200 mg

Phosphorus: 20 mg
Protein: 1 g
Calories: 60

Vegetable Crudité with Yogurt Dip

Ingredients:
1 carrot, cut into sticks
1 cucumber, sliced
1 bell pepper, sliced
1/2 cup low-fat Greek yogurt
1 tablespoon lemon juice
1 teaspoon chopped dill
Salt and pepper to taste

Preparation:
Arrange carrot sticks, cucumber slices, and bell pepper slices on a plate.
In a small bowl, mix together low-fat Greek yogurt, lemon juice, chopped dill, salt, and pepper to make the dip.
Serve the vegetable crudité with the yogurt dip.
Nutritional Information (per serving):
Sodium: 50 mg
Potassium: 200 mg
Phosphorus: 60 mg
Protein: 6 g
Calories: 70

Stuffed Celery Sticks

Ingredients:
4 celery stalks, cut into sticks
1/4 cup low-fat cream cheese

1 tablespoon chopped walnuts
1 tablespoon raisins
Pinch of cinnamon

Preparation:
In a small bowl, mix together low-fat cream cheese, chopped walnuts, raisins, and cinnamon.
Fill each celery stick with the cream cheese mixture.
Serve chilled.
Nutritional Information (per serving):
Sodium: 80 mg
Potassium: 150 mg
Phosphorus: 40 mg
Protein: 2 g
Calories: 60

Tuna Salad Lettuce Wraps

Ingredients:
1 can (5 oz) tuna, drained
2 tablespoons plain Greek yogurt
1 tablespoon diced red onion
1 tablespoon diced celery
1 tablespoon diced pickles
Salt and pepper to taste
Lettuce leaves, for wrapping

Preparation:
In a bowl, mix together tuna, plain Greek yogurt, diced red onion, diced celery, diced pickles, salt, and pepper.
Spoon the tuna salad onto lettuce leaves.
Wrap the lettuce leaves around the tuna salad.
Serve immediately.

Nutritional Information (per serving):
Sodium: 200 mg
Potassium: 250 mg
Phosphorus: 150 mg
Protein: 20 g
Calories: 150

Quinoa and Vegetable Stuffed Bell Peppers

Ingredients:
2 bell peppers, halved and seeded
1/2 cup cooked quinoa
1/4 cup diced tomatoes
1/4 cup diced zucchini
1/4 cup diced mushrooms
1 tablespoon olive oil
1/2 teaspoon dried oregano
Salt and pepper to taste

Preparation:
Preheat oven to 375°F (190°C).
In a skillet, heat olive oil over medium heat.
Sauté diced zucchini and mushrooms until tender.
Add cooked quinoa, diced tomatoes, dried oregano, salt, and pepper to the skillet. Cook until heated through.
Stuff bell pepper halves with the quinoa and vegetable mixture.
Bake in the preheated oven for 20-25 minutes until peppers are tender.
Nutritional Information (per serving):
Sodium: 40 mg
Potassium: 200 mg
Phosphorus: 100 mg

Protein: 5 g
Calories: 120

Cottage Cheese with Pineapple

Ingredients:
1/2 cup low-fat cottage cheese
1/2 cup diced pineapple
1 tablespoon chopped almonds
1 teaspoon honey (optional)

Preparation:
In a bowl, combine low-fat cottage cheese and diced pineapple.
Sprinkle chopped almonds on top.
Drizzle with honey (if using) for added sweetness.
Nutritional Information (per serving):
Sodium: 250 mg
Potassium: 200 mg
Phosphorus: 150 mg
Protein: 15 g
Calories: 140

Spinach and Feta Stuffed Mushrooms

Ingredients:
6 large mushrooms, stems removed
1 cup chopped spinach
1/4 cup crumbled feta cheese
1 tablespoon olive oil
1 clove garlic, minced
Salt and pepper to taste

Preparation:
Preheat oven to 375°F (190°C).
In a skillet, heat olive oil over medium heat.
Sauté minced garlic until fragrant.
Add chopped spinach and cook until wilted.
Remove from heat and stir in crumbled feta cheese, salt, and pepper.
Stuff mushroom caps with the spinach and feta mixture.
Bake in the preheated oven for 15-20 minutes until mushrooms are tender.
Nutritional Information (per serving):
Sodium: 70 mg
Potassium: 300 mg
Phosphorus: 100 mg
Protein: 5 g
Calories: 70

Apple Slices with Almond Butter

Ingredients:
1 apple, sliced
2 tablespoons almond butter (unsweetened)

Preparation:
Spread almond butter on apple slices.
Serve immediately.
Nutritional Information (per serving):
Sodium: 0 mg
Potassium: 200 mg
Phosphorus: 50 mg
Protein: 3 g
Calories: 120

Oatmeal Raisin Energy Bites

Ingredients:
1 cup rolled oats
1/4 cup almond butter (unsweetened)
1/4 cup honey (or maple syrup)
1/4 cup raisins
1/4 teaspoon cinnamon
Pinch of salt

Preparation:
In a bowl, mix together rolled oats, almond butter, honey (or maple syrup), raisins, cinnamon, and salt until well combined.
Roll the mixture into small balls.
Place energy bites on a parchment-lined baking sheet and refrigerate for at least 30 minutes to firm up.
Serve chilled.
Nutritional Information (per serving):
Sodium: 10 mg
Potassium: 100 mg
Phosphorus: 60 mg
Protein: 3 g
Calories: 100

Smoothies Recipes

Berry Blast Smoothie

Ingredients:

1/2 cup mixed berries (such as strawberries, blueberries, and raspberries)
1/2 banana
1/2 cup low-fat Greek yogurt
1/2 cup unsweetened almond milk
1 tablespoon honey (optional)

Preparation:
Combine mixed berries, banana, low-fat Greek yogurt, and unsweetened almond milk in a blender.
Blend until smooth.
Add honey if desired for extra sweetness.
Pour into a glass and serve immediately.
Nutritional Information (per serving):
Sodium: 50 mg
Potassium: 300 mg
Phosphorus: 100 mg
Protein: 8 g
Calories: 150

Green Goddess Smoothie

Ingredients:
1 cup spinach leaves
1/2 cucumber, peeled and chopped
1/2 green apple, cored and chopped
1/2 cup pineapple chunks
1/2 cup coconut water (unsweetened)

Preparation:
Combine spinach leaves, cucumber, green apple, pineapple chunks, and coconut water in a blender.
Blend until smooth.
Pour into a glass and serve immediately.

Nutritional Information (per serving):
Sodium: 60 mg
Potassium: 400 mg
Phosphorus: 80 mg
Protein: 3 g
Calories: 90

Banana Almond Smoothie

Ingredients:
1 ripe banana
1 tablespoon almond butter (unsweetened)
1/2 cup low-fat Greek yogurt
1/2 cup unsweetened almond milk
1 teaspoon honey (optional)

Preparation:
In a blender, combine ripe banana, almond butter, low-fat Greek yogurt, and unsweetened almond milk.
Blend until smooth.
Add honey if desired for sweetness.
Pour into a glass and serve immediately.
Nutritional Information (per serving):
Sodium: 70 mg
Potassium: 400 mg
Phosphorus: 100 mg
Protein: 7 g
Calories: 180

Tropical Paradise Smoothie

Ingredients:
1/2 cup mango chunks

1/2 cup pineapple chunks
1/2 banana
1/2 cup low-fat coconut milk
1/2 cup unsweetened almond milk

Preparation:
Combine mango chunks, pineapple chunks, banana, low-fat coconut milk, and unsweetened almond milk in a blender.
Blend until smooth.
Pour into a glass and serve immediately.
Nutritional Information (per serving):
Sodium: 40 mg
Potassium: 350 mg
Phosphorus: 90 mg
Protein: 3 g
Calories: 140

Berry Spinach Protein Smoothie

Ingredients:
1/2 cup mixed berries (such as strawberries, blueberries, and raspberries)
1/2 cup spinach leaves
1/2 cup low-fat Greek yogurt
1/2 cup unsweetened almond milk
1 scoop vanilla protein powder (low phosphorus)

Preparation:

Combine mixed berries, spinach leaves, low-fat Greek yogurt, unsweetened almond milk, and vanilla protein powder in a blender.
Blend until smooth.
Pour into a glass and serve immediately.
Nutritional Information (per serving):
Sodium: 60 mg
Potassium: 300 mg
Phosphorus: 120 mg
Protein: 20 g
Calories: 200

Peachy Keen Smoothie

Ingredients:
1 ripe peach, pitted and chopped
1/2 banana
1/2 cup low-fat Greek yogurt
1/2 cup unsweetened almond milk
1 tablespoon chia seeds

Preparation:
Combine ripe peach, banana, low-fat Greek yogurt, unsweetened almond milk, and chia seeds in a blender.
Blend until smooth.
Pour into a glass and serve immediately.
Nutritional Information (per serving):
Sodium: 50 mg
Potassium: 350 mg
Phosphorus: 100 mg
Protein: 8 g
Calories: 160

Cherry Vanilla Smoothie

Ingredients:
1/2 cup pitted cherries (fresh or frozen)
1/2 cup low-fat Greek yogurt
1/2 cup unsweetened almond milk
1/4 teaspoon vanilla extract
1 teaspoon honey (optional)

Preparation:
Combine pitted cherries, low-fat Greek yogurt, unsweetened almond milk, vanilla extract, and honey (if using) in a blender.
Blend until smooth.
Pour into a glass and serve immediately.
Nutritional Information (per serving):
Sodium: 40 mg
Potassium: 300 mg
Phosphorus: 80 mg
Protein: 8 g
Calories: 150

Minty Pineapple Smoothie

Ingredients:
1/2 cup pineapple chunks
1/2 banana
1/2 cup spinach leaves
1/2 cup low-fat Greek yogurt
1/2 cup unsweetened almond milk
Handful of fresh mint leaves

Preparation:
Combine pineapple chunks, banana, spinach leaves, low-fat Greek yogurt, unsweetened almond milk, and fresh mint leaves in a blender.
Blend until smooth.
Pour into a glass and serve immediately.
Nutritional Information (per serving):
Sodium: 60 mg
Potassium: 350 mg
Phosphorus: 90 mg
Protein: 7 g
Calories: 150

Carrot Cake Smoothie

Ingredients:
1/2 cup grated carrot
1/2 banana
1/4 cup rolled oats
1/2 cup low-fat Greek yogurt
1/2 cup unsweetened almond milk
1/4 teaspoon ground cinnamon
1/4 teaspoon vanilla extract
Preparation:
Combine grated carrot, banana, rolled oats, low-fat Greek yogurt, unsweetened almond milk, ground cinnamon, and vanilla extract in a blender.
Blend until smooth.
Pour into a glass and serve immediately.
Nutritional Information (per serving):
Sodium: 60 mg
Potassium: 300 mg
Phosphorus: 80 mg

Protein: 7 g
Calories: 160

Citrus Sunshine Smoothie

Ingredients:
1/2 cup orange segments
1/2 cup pineapple chunks
1/2 banana
1/2 cup low-fat Greek yogurt
1/2 cup unsweetened almond milk

Preparation:
Combine orange segments, pineapple chunks, banana, low-fat Greek yogurt, and unsweetened almond milk in a blender.
Blend until smooth.
Pour into a glass and serve immediately.
Nutritional Information (per serving):
Sodium: 50 mg
Potassium: 350 mg
Phosphorus: 80 mg
Protein: 7 g
Calories: 140

Chocolate Peanut Butter Smoothie

Ingredients:
1 tablespoon cocoa powder (unsweetened)
1 tablespoon peanut butter (unsweetened)
1/2 banana
1/2 cup low-fat Greek yogurt
1/2 cup unsweetened almond milk

Preparation:
Combine cocoa powder, peanut butter, banana, low-fat Greek yogurt, and unsweetened almond milk in a blender. Blend until smooth.
Pour into a glass and serve immediately.
Nutritional Information (per serving):
Sodium: 70 mg
Potassium: 300 mg
Phosphorus: 100 mg
Protein: 8 g
Calories: 180

Vanilla Berry Smoothie

Ingredients:
1/2 cup mixed berries (such as strawberries, blueberries, and raspberries)
1/2 cup low-fat Greek yogurt
1/2 cup unsweetened almond milk
1/4 teaspoon vanilla extract
1 teaspoon honey (optional)

Preparation:
Combine mixed berries, low-fat Greek yogurt, unsweetened almond milk, vanilla extract, and honey (if using) in a blender.
Blend until smooth.
Pour into a glass and serve immediately.
Nutritional Information (per serving):
Sodium: 50 mg
Potassium: 300 mg

Phosphorus: 80 mg
Protein: 8 g
Calories: 150

Mango Coconut Smoothie

Ingredients:
1/2 cup mango chunks
1/2 banana
1/2 cup low-fat coconut milk
1/2 cup unsweetened almond milk
1 tablespoon shredded coconut (unsweetened)

Preparation:
Combine mango chunks, banana, low-fat coconut milk, unsweetened almond milk, and shredded coconut in a blender.
Blend until smooth.
Pour into a glass and serve immediately.
Nutritional Information (per serving):
Sodium: 40 mg
Potassium: 350 mg
Phosphorus: 90 mg
Protein: 3 g
Calories: 140

Pomegranate Blueberry Smoothie

Ingredients:
1/2 cup pomegranate seeds
1/2 cup blueberries (fresh or frozen)
1/2 banana
1/2 cup low-fat Greek yogurt
1/2 cup unsweetened almond milk

Preparation:
Combine pomegranate seeds, blueberries, banana, low-fat Greek yogurt, and unsweetened almond milk in a blender.
Blend until smooth.
Pour into a glass and serve immediately.
Nutritional Information (per serving):
Sodium: 60 mg
Potassium: 300 mg
Phosphorus: 80 mg
Protein: 7 g
Calories: 140

Avocado Kale Smoothie

Ingredients:
1/2 ripe avocado
1 cup chopped kale leaves
1/2 cup pineapple chunks
1/2 cup low-fat Greek yogurt
1/2 cup unsweetened almond milk

Preparation:
Combine ripe avocado, chopped kale leaves, pineapple chunks, low-fat Greek yogurt, and unsweetened almond milk in a blender.
Blend until smooth.
Pour into a glass and serve immediately.
Nutritional Information (per serving):
Sodium: 60 mg

Potassium: 400 mg
Phosphorus: 100 mg
Protein: 7 g
Calories: 170

BONUS
Shopping list

Produce:

1. Spinach
2. Kale
3. Swiss chard
4. Romaine lettuce
5. Bell peppers (various colors)
6. Cucumbers
7. Tomatoes
8. Carrots
9. Celery
10. Zucchini
11. Squash (summer and winter varieties)
12. Broccoli
13. Cauliflower
14. Green beans
15. Asparagus
16. Brussel sprouts
17. Onions
18. Garlic
19. Shallots
20. Leeks
21. Mushrooms
22. Avocados

23. Lemons
24. Limes
25. Oranges
26. Apples
27. Berries (strawberries, blueberries, raspberries)
28. Bananas
29. Mangoes
30. Pineapple
31. Papaya
32. Kiwi
33. Grapes
34. Peaches
35. Plums
36. Pears
37. Pomegranate seeds
38. Dates
39. Figs
40. Raisins

Dairy and Alternatives:

1. Low-fat Greek yogurt
2. Low-fat cottage cheese
3. Unsweetened almond milk
4. Unsweetened coconut milk
5. Low-fat cheese (mozzarella, feta)
6. Eggs

Protein Sources:

1. Skinless chicken breasts
2. Turkey breast
3. Fish (salmon, cod, tilapia)
4. Shrimp

5. Tofu
6. Tempeh
7. Seitan
8. Canned tuna (in water)
9. Canned salmon (in water)
10. Canned beans (kidney beans, black beans, chickpeas)
11. Lentils
12. Split peas

Grains and Starches:

1. Quinoa
2. Brown rice
3. Wild rice
4. Barley
5. Bulgur
6. Millet
7. Oats
8. Whole wheat pasta
9. Whole grain bread
10. Whole grain tortillas

Nuts, Seeds, and Nut Butters:

1. Almonds
2. Walnuts
3. Pecans
4. Cashews

5. Pistachios
6. Chia seeds
7. Flaxseeds
8. Sunflower seeds
9. Pumpkin seeds
10. Natural peanut butter
11. Almond butter

Fats and Oils:

1. Olive oil
2. Avocado oil
3. Coconut oil
4. Flaxseed oil

Herbs and Spices:

1. Basil
2. Parsley
3. Cilantro
4. Dill
5. Mint
6. Thyme
7. Rosemary
8. Oregano
9. Paprika
10. Cumin
11. Turmeric
12. Ginger
13. Garlic powder
14. Onion powder
15. Cayenne pepper
16. Black pepper
17. Sea salt (in moderation)

Condiments and Flavorings:

1. Mustard (low-sodium)
2. Vinegar (balsamic, apple cider, red wine)
3. Low-sodium soy sauce or tamari
4. Hot sauce (without added sodium)
5. Salsa (low-sodium)
6. Tomato paste (no added salt)
7. Low-sodium broth or bouillon cubes
8. Unsweetened cocoa powder
9. Vanilla extract
10. Lemon juice

Canned and Packaged Goods:

1. Canned low-sodium beans
2. Canned diced tomatoes (no added salt)
3. Canned coconut milk (unsweetened)
4. Whole grain cereal (low-sugar)
5. Whole grain crackers (low-sodium)
6. Rice cakes (low-sodium)
7. Popcorn kernels (for air-popping)

Frozen Foods:

1. Frozen mixed vegetables (no added sauce)
2. Frozen berries (unsweetened)
3. Frozen spinach
4. Frozen cauliflower rice

Beverages:

1. Filtered water
2. Herbal teas (caffeine-free)

3. Unsweetened fruit juices (limit intake)

Sweeteners:

1. Honey (in moderation)
2. Maple syrup (in moderation)
3. Stevia (in moderation)

Miscellaneous:

1. Low-sodium baking powder
2. Low-sodium baking soda
3. Low-sodium marinades and sauces
4. Low-sodium salad dressings
5. Low-sodium seasoning blends
6. Low-sodium vegetable juice
7. Low-sodium canned soup (if needed)

Kitchen Staples:

1. Aluminum foil
2. Parchment paper
3. Plastic wrap
4. Zip-top bags (various sizes)
5. Food storage containers
6. Cooking spray

Health and Wellness:

1. Multivitamin (specifically formulated for kidney health)
2. Mineral supplements (as recommended by healthcare provider)
3. Kidney-friendly protein powder (if needed)

Medical Supplies:

1. Blood pressure monitor
2. Blood glucose monitor (if needed)
3. Insulin (if needed)
4. Prescription medications (as prescribed)

Personal Care:

1. Hand soap
2. Hand sanitizer
3. Dishwashing detergent
4. Laundry detergent

Household Supplies:

1. Toilet paper
2. Paper towels
3. Cleaning supplies (all-purpose cleaner, disinfectant spray)

Specialty Items (Optional):

1. Low-sodium baking mixes
2. Kidney-friendly cookbooks
3. Meal planning tools (such as portion control containers)

4. Food scale
5. Blender or food processor
6. Air fryer
7. Slow cooker or Instant Pot
8. Non-stick cookware

Note:
1. Always check food labels for sodium, potassium, and phosphorus content.
2. Choose fresh or frozen fruits and vegetables over canned varieties when possible to reduce sodium intake.
3. Drink water or other kidney-friendly beverages throughout the day to stay hydrated.
4. Limit intake of processed and packaged foods high in sodium, potassium, and phosphorus.

CONCLUSION

As we reach the end of the Kidney Disease Diet Cookbook for Women, it's important to reflect on the journey we've taken together and the invaluable insights we've gained along the way. This cookbook was crafted with a singular purpose: to empower women living with kidney disease to take charge of their health through mindful dietary choices and delicious, kidney-friendly recipes.

Throughout these pages, we've delved into the intricate nuances of kidney health, exploring the anatomy and function of the kidneys, understanding common types and causes of kidney disease, recognizing early symptoms, identifying risk factors, and implementing proactive prevention strategies. We've also navigated the complexities of a kidney-friendly diet, from managing sodium intake to balancing potassium and phosphorus levels, and everything in between.

But beyond the nutritional aspects, this cookbook is a testament to the resilience, strength, and determination of women facing the challenges of kidney disease. It's a celebration of the power of food to heal, nourish, and uplift both body and spirit. Each recipe is a labor of love, meticulously crafted to provide not only sustenance but also joy and satisfaction.

As women, i understand the importance of self-care and self-compassion. Living with kidney disease may present its own set of obstacles, but it also offers an opportunity for growth, resilience, and empowerment. By embracing a kidney-friendly lifestyle, we honor our bodies, our health, and our well-being.

As you continue your journey towards optimal kidney health, remember that you are not alone. You have a community of support behind you, cheering you on every step of the way. And within the pages of this cookbook, you have a treasure trove of recipes, tips, and resources to guide you on your path.

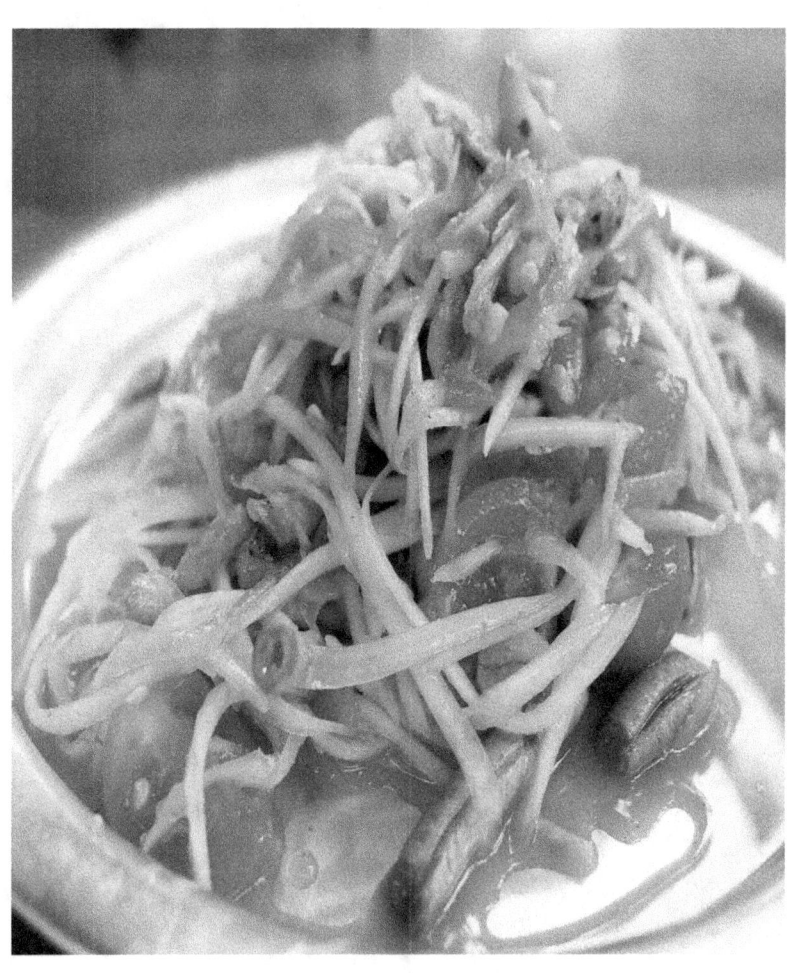

www.ingramcontent.com/pod-product-compliance
Lightning Source LLC
Chambersburg PA
CBHW071054240526
45471CB00015B/1876